THE
POWER
METER
HANDBOOK

THE
POWER
METER
HANDBOOK

A User's Guide for Cyclists and Triathletes

BY JOE FRIEL

Boulder, Colorado

3002 Sterling Circle, Suite 100
Boulder, Colorado 80301-2338 USA
(303) 440-0601 · Fax (303) 444-6788 · E-mail velopress@competitorgroup.com

Distributed in the United States and Canada by Ingram Publisher Services

A Cataloging-in-Publication record for this book is available from the Library of Congress.
ISBN 978-1-934030-95-0

For information on purchasing VeloPress books, please call (800) 811-4210, ext. 2138, or visit www.velopress.com.

Cover and interior design by Heidi Carcella
Cover photograph by Brad Kaminski; screen image courtesy of CycleOps
Power chart illustrations adapted by Charles Chamberlin

Text set in Minion Pro

12   13   14 / 10   9   8   7   6   5   4   3   2   1

CONTENTS

PART III How Can I Use My Power Meter to Improve My
Competitive Performance?

PART I

WHAT IS A POWER METER, AND HOW CAN IT HELP ME?

Why Use a Power Meter?

WHY DO YOU TRAIN? Before you answer that question, I want to make sure we're talking about the same thing. You will come across the words "train" and "training" often in this book. They are common in an athlete's vocabulary. What I mean when using them here is *working out with a purpose.* That purpose is to improve performance. In this book, performance has to do with a bike-related event, such as a triathlon, road race, time trial, mountain bike race, or century ride.

Let's drill down a little deeper. By "performance," I'm talking about riding competitively—preparing to become fitter and therefore faster in order to improve on your previous results in similar events or to finish high in your event category. Some athletes compete with others, while some compete only with themselves by trying to improve on previous performances. Either is fine. Both require purposeful workouts to produce greater fitness.

If the workout purpose is *not* bike performance—if, for example, it's losing weight or improving health, both of which are worthy goals—then it's exercise, not training, to my way of thinking. Power meters can be useful for any of these desired results. But the purpose we'll be examining in great detail here is training—purposeful workouts intended to produce better event performance.

The power meter is a powerful tool for training, one that can potentially make you fitter and faster than any other piece of equipment you could get for your bike. Even if you have been in the sport for a long time and achieved all the fitness you think is possible, I guarantee that you have room for improvement. I've coached athletes who have gone from years of middle-of-the-pack finishes to the podium within one season after starting to train with a power meter. I'm certain you can, also. The upper limit of potential for performance in sport is remarkably high and largely untapped by almost all athletes. This is where a power meter can make a difference.

You may know of someone who has a power meter but has never really seen any significant improvement in performance because of it. That's common. Power meters are not magic. You don't just put one on your bike and all of a sudden become faster. When you begin using one for the first time, it looks simple enough—just a number on your handlebars that changes as you go harder or easier. And you might find yourself thinking, "What's the big deal?" I've heard that from new power meter owners a lot. "The numbers are interesting, but so what?" It's not until you begin to look at the downloaded data with your computer software that the magic happens—if you know what all the numbers mean. If you've looked at the data after a ride, then you know what I'm talking about. It can be a bit overwhelming. That ever-changing flow of numbers you saw on your handlebars during the ride has somehow morphed into graphs, tables, and charts. What does it all mean? How is it going to make you fitter and faster?

For now you're just going to have to take my word that it will. But after reading and applying the basic concepts in this book, you'll see change. Your new power meter will help you become a better rider. We'll get into the details of how to do that in subsequent chapters. First, let's look at what the power meter can do to improve your performance and why it's better than any other training tool.

WHY POWER?

To become fitter and faster, you need to make physical and perhaps even mental changes as you prepare for an event. Your power meter can help you do both. Here are five performance-enhancing ways that a power meter can improve your training once you know how to use it.

Make Training Precisely Match the Demands of the Race

This is undoubtedly the most important reason for using a power meter. Effective training demands precision for you to become more fit. The obvious question is "Fit for what?" Every high-performance event, whether it's a 6-hour Ironman® triathlon ride or a 45-minute criterium, demands a specific type of fitness. This comes down to getting the duration and intensity of the key workouts right. Duration is easy. A stopwatch or an odometer will do. But intensity is a different story and raises some very important issues for your training.

The first intensity issue has to do with the specific demands of the goal event. How intense—in other words, how hard—will it be? Some events, the 6-hour Ironman ride, for example, require you to put out a steady but relatively low intensity for a long time. In contrast, the 45-minute criterium race fluctuates between extremely high and low intensities. Training with the same intensity for both of these events simply won't work. Your key workouts must reflect the exact levels of intensity demanded by the event in order for you to become fit for it.

Without a power meter, you're just guessing at how hard to make your key workouts. If you guess wrong—either too high or too low—you'll have a poor performance. With a power meter, you'll know exactly what the intensity demands of the event are so that you can replicate them in training. Then over the course of a few weeks, you can make your workouts increasingly like the goal event by training at the precise intensities needed. On race day there will be no surprises. Your body will be ready to meet the demands of the event.

Pace Steady-State Races

To be successful in steady-state events such as time trials and triathlons, you must expend your energy in a well-calculated manner. This is called "pacing." It's hard to get right, even for seasoned veterans of the sport. Most go out much too fast at the start and pay the price in the second half of the race by significantly slowing down. This is the most common mistake made in steady-state events. I see it happen in every race. It can be easily fixed with a power meter in a much more precise manner than with a heart rate monitor. In fact, your heart rate monitor is probably setting you up for poor race pacing. (You may be shaking your head at that idea, but it's true. I'll come back to it later in this chapter to explain why.)

Proper pacing goes well beyond the common problem of going out too fast at the start. It also has to do with energy expenditure on hills, including tiny ones; in headwinds and tailwinds; and over the entire course so that you finish strong. You will learn in Chapter 4 how your power meter makes this simple.

Know and Increase Your Limits

There is a similar problem, but with a twist, if you do variably paced races such as criteriums, road races, and mountain bike races. Here the challenge is that other riders often dictate your pacing strategy. There are brief episodes, such as breakaways, sprints, and aggressive hill climbs, in these types of races that often determine the outcome. They usually last less than two minutes but are critical moments. If for these episodes you are able to stay with the leaders, then you will make the "selection" and can place well, perhaps even win.

The key is knowing what to expect in regard to the intensity, duration, and frequency of these episodes. Armed with a typical race power profile from similar races, you will know exactly what you are currently capable of doing when they occur—and better yet, you can train to respond to them. You can even train to eventually become the rider who initiates them, putting the hurt on others. We'll discuss these concepts in much greater detail in Chapter 4.

Organize Your Season

Planning your race season is called "periodization." You're probably familiar with the concept since it's been around since the 1960s and is still used by nearly all elite athletes around the world. I wrote about it in some detail in my Training Bible book series. In a nutshell, periodization involves manipulating training volume and intensity to produce high levels of fitness at times in the season when you have important races—what I term "A-priority." With a power meter, you can use something called "Training Stress Score"™ to organize your season around A-priority races. This method is much more precise than using weekly hours or miles and estimates of intensity. We'll get into this in Chapter 7.

Measure Fitness Changes

There are two questions athletes want answered throughout the season. The first and most basic is "Am I becoming fitter and faster?" The second is "How do I compare with my competition?" The "competition" could be you from the same race the previous year, or it could be the other athletes whom you expect to show up. The answers give you insight into what to expect in a race. With your power meter, you can answer both. I'll show you how in Chapter 6.

Other Power Meter Benefits

The five benefits I list above are just the beginning. There are many more that will be discussed throughout the book, including the following:

- Setting specific goals that relate directly to your desired race performances
- Using personal power zones to train effectively
- Measuring performance progress
- Peaking for races with a plan for coming into "form" at the right times
- Quantifying fatigue and understanding how to manage it
- Knowing how many calories you expend in a workout or race so that you can focus on nutritional recovery
- Improving your efficiency by comparing power and heart rate
- Communicating better with your coach regarding what you've done in workouts and races
- Motivating you to train harder (I sometimes have to hold back the athletes I coach who become overly excited about what they see happening when first using a power meter)
- Achieving peak race performances

The bottom line is that learning how to train with power will improve your training and your racing. But the benefits won't come if you are unwilling to change the way you train. If you've been training by "feel" for a long time and are stuck in one way of doing it, you are unlikely to tap the many benefits of power-based training. There is no growth without change, and what you're about to learn will certainly require you to change your training perceptions. If you are unwilling to do that, then a power meter is not going to do you any good.

In contrast, I've seen significant and at times astounding changes in performance in the many athletes whom I've coached over the past decade since I started requiring them to have power meters. All of them improved. Some went from finishing well behind the leaders to standing at podiums in a short time. This never happened before they got power meters installed on their bikes and started using them as I'll describe in the following chapters. I'm sure doing so can make a big difference for you, also.

WHY NOT HEART RATE, SPEED, OR FEEL?

Why use a power meter? You've spent a wad of money to get one, and all you have to show for it so far are a fluctuating number on your handlebars and some software that looks pretty confusing. And, even worse, you apparently are going to have to change the way you train because of it. Why not just keep using heart rate, as you've been doing for years? You've come a long way in the sport by doing so. Or how about just using speed? What you're after, obviously, is simply to go faster. Handlebar computers with speedometers are cheap in comparison to both power and heart rate devices. So why not just use one of those? Or perhaps you are really old school and don't like anything on your bike displaying numbers. You just want to ride and race by feel. I know where you're coming from, as I've answered these questions for years. Let's take a brief look at why power is better if you want to perform at a higher level.

Heart Rate

Contrary to what most athletes believe, heart rate is reactive, not proactive. In other words, it responds to what the muscles are doing. It does not cause the muscles to work any harder. It's not the "engine"—it's simply the "fuel pump." When the engine (muscles) works harder going up a hill, the heart responds by pumping more blood to help the muscles keep going. Training based only on heart rate is like using the fuel gauge on your car to determine how fast you're driving. That can be done, but it's "bass-ackwards."

Now, don't get me wrong. The fuel pump (your heart) is quite valuable to performance. The engine (your muscles) couldn't work without it. How hard the pump is working is good information to know as it's indirectly related to performance. If the engine is demanding lots of fuel, then something hard is probably happening. So the pump had better be capable of delivering. But no race-car driver would use the fuel pump as a way of determining performance. The engine is at the center of fast car racing. The fuel pump is of secondary importance at best.

In the same way, we as bike racers are better off looking at what the engine is producing rather than at how hard the pump is working. In fact, your training should be focused on building the engine—your muscles. Contrary to what athletes who use heart rate monitors believe, muscle is where nearly all fitness changes take place. Focusing only on the rate at which blood is pumped to the muscles is not the most effective way to train.

More than likely you have been using a heart rate monitor ever since you started in your sport. They've been around since the late 1970s, so athletes have become quite used to them. And they've measurably helped to improve performance for many. But other than the pump-engine relationship I described above, there are still significant limitations to heart rate–based training. Heart rate is affected by "outside" forces, such as diet, race-day excitement, and psychological stress. For example, caffeinated drinks and even a shot of sugar can cause heart rate to rise regardless of how hard you are pushing yourself. Simply being around other riders, especially in a race, will also result in an artificially high heart rate. And even the stuff that goes on between your ears—an argument with the boss, tax time, and other worries—has an effect on heart rate that is unrelated to your riding intensity. Furthermore, in training heart rate is slow to respond when you are doing intervals, so during the first few minutes of each interval you are forced to guess how hard to go. All of this sets you up for poor workout and race pacing. It could very well be the reason you've not done as well as you are capable of doing, especially in steady-paced racing such as time trials and triathlons.

Still, the greatest limitation is that heart rate doesn't tell you anything about how you are performing. It only tells you, indirectly, how hard the engine is working based on the engine's demand for fuel and oxygen. To be truly effective, heart rate must be compared with something else. I will show you in Chapter 6 how power and heart rate can be compared and how the benefits of this relationship can be useful for your training.

Speed

Several years ago, I was invited to go for a long Saturday-morning ride with a couple of Ironman triathletes who were in their final stages of race preparation. They didn't have power meters. We rolled out of the parking lot, and they immediately increased their speed to about 25 mph and held it there. There was no warm-up or conversation. We were immediately riding all out. After several minutes of this, I rode up next to one of them and asked what was going on. Why so fast? He told me that they wanted to average 22 mph and knew that because of hills and the possibility of wind, they had to get the average speed high when they were still fresh. After a couple of hours, the ride slowed to a death march as fatigue set in. They didn't quite achieve their speed goal that day, which meant they'd have to go out faster at the start on the following weekend. What a strange way of training.

Speed on a bicycle is largely determined by wind and hills. If you're riding uphill or into a strong headwind, you're going slow. Downhill and with a tailwind, you're riding fast. Whatever my riding companions' average speed was at the end of the workout would have to be explained based on the environmental conditions, not their fitness. Was it a windy day? How hard was the wind blowing when they rode into or with it? Were they going uphill or downhill? How steep were the hills? How great would the wind speed be on race day? Would there be a tailwind or a headwind on the longest hill of the race? There is absolutely no way of estimating performance requirements and preparing to be ready for them if speed is the measure of intensity.

With a power meter, hills and wind are of no consequence. In a race, while others are guessing how fast to ride up hills and into the wind, the rider with a power meter is content simply holding the prescribed power. Power is a much easier and much more precise measure of intensity than speed.

Feel

I recently received a comment from a rider after I posted a blog entry called "Why You Need a Power Meter." He told me he trained with an elite cyclist who didn't use a power meter, a heart rate monitor, or even a handlebar computer with a speedometer. And his friend was really fit and fast. So he now believed that riding based strictly on how he feels is the proper way to train. Sport scientists call this method of training "perceived exertion." They use scales to rate this, such as 0 to 10, with 10 being high. By assigning a number to how hard the effort feels, they create a subjective quantifying system known as "rating of perceived exertion" (RPE).

Actually, there's a lot to be said for that way of thinking. If the battery on your power meter or whatever device you use dies on race day, you had better be able to continue on without it and still race effectively. Racing by feel, or RPE, is the way all riders did it in the early part of the previous century.

The elite rider mentioned above is undoubtedly what I call an "artist-athlete." Elites usually fall into this category. Artist-athletes despise numbers because they "get in the way of *real* racing." That's the way artists think regardless of the medium. Their actions are totally subjective. They just seemed like the right thing to do at the time.

There are many nonelites who down deep are artist-athletes and would really like to race based strictly on feel. Some can do it successfully. But not all athletes are good at doing so, as riding by feel requires a calm, focused approach to the race. Most of us race based on emotions. We start too fast because we're excited, and eventually we blow up. The same thing happens when we do training rides, such as tempo, intervals, hill repeats, or anything else requiring patience and precision: We start out too fast and then fade. We need a device of some sort—a power meter or even a heart rate monitor—to teach us what the proper intensity feels like. Once that knowledge of proper intensity is eventually drilled in, racing by feel becomes possible.

Another type of athlete is the "scientist-athlete." These athletes train to improve performance by trying personal experiments and measuring outcomes so that they can find what works best for them. If you're one of these, you'll thrive with a power meter, as it's probably the best tool there is for science experiments on cyclists.

Some people are a mix of artist and scientist. Lance Armstrong is an example. In his prime he liked to experiment and precisely measure everything in training, from calories consumed to wind drag over clothing to power with different bike designs. But when it came to racing, he was an artist who could fool competitors by acting fatigued or blowing them away on a climb after an angry glance.

You probably know by now which type of athlete you tend to be. Unless you have training and racing by feel totally figured out and are at the peak of your potential, which is doubtful, I feel certain that a power meter can help you. I've seen that happen with every athlete, regardless of type, whom I have ever coached with a power-based program.

Multisystem Training

From what you've just read, you may think I'm advising you to disregard your heart rate, speed, and RPE. I'm not. Each is important in its own way and should be monitored throughout a ride. It's just that looking at the ride through the lens of power makes better sense of all that you are seeing and experiencing from the other three; it makes them more relevant. With power you see the world of training more completely than ever before. It's like the difference between watching a movie in 3D and watching it only in 2D. In 3D, everything is clearer and more meaningful.

Figure 1.1 illustrates my point. It shows what happens in regard to heart rate, RPE, speed, and power while a rider is steadily climbing a hill, coasting down the other side, and then starting to pedal again on flat terrain.

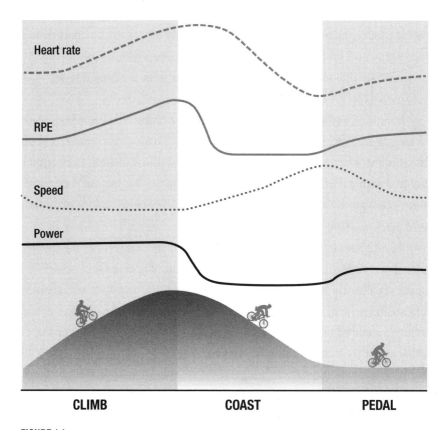

FIGURE 1.1 The responses of heart rate, rating of perceived exertion (RPE), speed, and power when climbing a hill, coasting down, and pedaling on flat terrain

Notice that heart rate and RPE rise as the hill is steadily climbed, while speed and power remain fairly constant. When the rider is coasting down the hill, speed increases as heart rate, RPE, and power decline. Note that heart rate is slow to respond as the rider starts up the hill, and heart rate continues to increase in the early part of the descent. This lag is common with heart rate. RPE increases on the climb as fatigue gradually sets in. RPE rather quickly decreases on the downhill side before rising again as pedaling is resumed on flat terrain. Speed remains constantly low on the uphill, increases on the descent, and eventually settles in at a steady rate with the return to flat terrain.

Now look at the power line. It reflects some of the changes taking place in the other three, but it does so rather quickly. Following a steady level on the climb, power almost immediately responds to the transition from climbing to coasting and from coasting to pedaling on the flat section. The power line presents the most useful picture of the athlete's performance because it is a direct measurement of the rider's output.

The higher the power is up the hill and on the flat terrain, the greater the rider's performance is. The same can be said of speed. Only power and speed are directly related to performance. Heart rate and RPE tell us nothing about performance—they simply reflect what the rider is experiencing. When compared with power, however, heart rate and RPE also tell us something about the rider's fitness. When power is high and heart rate and RPE are relatively low compared with previous rides on that same hill, we know that the athlete is fitter and faster.

OUTPUT AND INPUT

There's an important point in the last paragraph that I want to make sure you got: "Only power and speed are directly related to performance. Heart rate and RPE tell us nothing about performance—they simply reflect what the rider is experiencing."

What I'm describing here are output and input. Power and speed are measures of output. They tell us what is being accomplished during a ride. Heart rate and RPE are input. They tell us what the effort is to create the output.

This is an important distinction. Races give out awards based on output—who got to the finish line first. There are no awards for input—who worked the hardest to get there. In fact, if everyone in a category is trying to win a typical race, input will be much the same across the entire field. Everyone will be working hard. Input will be high. But despite that, only one person will come across the finish line first. That person will have had the highest output.

Both factors are important, but only one produces actual results. In Chapter 6 I'll show you how the relationship between output and input is an important indicator for your training.

WARNING!

Power meters are not perfect. There are definite downsides to training with power. (Sounds odd in a book on power meters, huh? Let me explain.)

I've already touched on one in the earlier portion titled "Feel." The "safety" bike (the successor to the "penny-farthing" bike with the huge front wheel) and bike racing, in whatever format, have been around since the late 19th century. Throughout most of that time, training and racing on a bike were almost entirely an art form. Athletes did whatever seemed right at the time based almost entirely on how they felt. They were magnificently in tune with their bodies. They had no choice.

Today, however, I'm afraid athletes may be losing their sense for the "art of racing." Bike-related sports have most decidedly become more science and less art in the past 30 years. This is probably true across the board in all sports, but especially in cycle sports. The heart rate monitor started this trend, but the power meter has taken it to a whole new level. Bicycle road races still demand a great reliance on feel and art since such races are largely unstructured, and the race circumstances and demands on the body change frequently as the race progresses. One of the only ways to develop a sense of feel and art is through racing itself, as races give us the best chance to experience those changing conditions.

Nevertheless, *training* for road races has very definitely become a science. Steady-state bike races, such as time trials and triathlons, and even mountain bike racing to some extent, are very close to becoming all science all the time.

This lament may sound strange coming from me since I am probably one of the strongest proponents of the science of training. But I feel a bit of a loss as athletes change the way they prepare for and compete in their sports.

Having a sense for the art of training and racing is a worthy trait that leads to greater insight into what your body is experiencing. I'm afraid that we may be losing that ability to some extent. To stave off that loss, it may be good for your total development as an athlete to occasionally—perhaps once a week—not have any numbers to look at during a ride or a portion of it. For these times, you can remove the handlebar computer and put it in your back pocket if it is wireless. That way you can still collect the data for later analysis to see how your "feel" for riding a bike is coming along. If your device is not wireless, put a piece of tape over the computer display.

This leads to my next warning. For some riders—mostly the scientist-athletes among us—numbers are addictive and even highly motivating. For them, training is all about producing numbers, especially high numbers. That's okay on days when training is meant to be challenging. But it's not such a good thing for recovery days. Trying to keep the numbers high for these workouts is counterproductive. If you find yourself fixated on maintaining your "fitness," even on easy days, then it's best to put the computer in your pocket or put tape on it. Just ride easy on those days without having a number associated with it other than RPE.

When you first start riding with a power meter, the handlebar readout can be captivating. There are lots of numbers, and they are constantly changing. It's easy to lose your focus on the road and the cars around you owing to your concentration on the display. Because of this, for your first few workouts with a power meter, ride where the traffic is light and there are few intersections. Once you get the hang of the meter, you can get back to your usual routes. But always ride with your focus primarily on what's going on around you rather than on what your power meter is displaying.

Despite this appeal to set aside your power meter once in a while so that you can concentrate on how your body feels and responds as you train, I want to emphasize once more that using your new device for *most* of your time on the bike has the potential to make you fitter and faster than ever before. Once you have a solid understanding of the basics of the meter's use, as I'll describe in later chapters, your performance will be greatly enhanced. That's the bottom line for *why* you should train with power. Now let's move on to *what* power is.

2

What Is Power?

I HOPE THAT CHAPTER 1 gave you a better understanding of why your power meter is such a valuable tool and why it is becoming so widely used by athletes in all bike-related sports. In this chapter I will explain *what* power is all about. I should warn you in advance that it will get a bit technical at times. But by the end of this chapter, you should be able to explain to your riding partners what your power meter is measuring and roughly how it does so. You should also be able to tell them how you're using it to get fitter and faster.

THE BASICS OF POWER

Let's start this discussion with the most common term used in power: the watt. On a power meter, we call the numbers displayed on the handlebar computer "watts." Watts indicate how much energy you're expending during the ride and, as you'll see below, how fast you're expending it. We'll come back to this relationship of power and energy in Chapter 6.

The unit of power is named after James Watt (1736–1819), a Scottish inventor and mechanical engineer. He was a genius who is credited with discovering in 1765 how to make the steam engine more powerful and efficient (exactly what we are after for your bike performance), thus making the Industrial Revolution of the late 18th and early 19th centuries possible. He also developed the concept of horsepower and formulated the fundamental mathematics for power measurement.

Power in Physics

To help us get a broader understanding of power, let's look at how physics describes it. After all, concepts about power arose in physics, and power—your individual power output, specifically—is the key to improving your cycling performance. Some of what follows may be a bit difficult to grasp on the first read, but hang in there with me as you think your way through this. In the end you'll have a deeper appreciation for what's going on when you ride your bike with a power meter. I'll try to make my explanation as simple and painless as possible. Here we go.

The watt is a measure of power determined by calculating the rate (think "time") at which work is done. By "work" I don't mean your job but rather the physical act of moving something, such as standing up while doing a squat exercise with a heavy barbell on your shoulders in the weight room. That's work. Work doesn't care whether you stand up on the squat fast or slow; you moved the weight from here to there, so the amount of work remains the same no matter how long you take to do it.

Power itself is how much work you are doing *and* how fast you are doing it. The faster you stand up (shortening the time of the movement), the more power you are producing on the squat. Physicists express this relationship of power, work, and time as a formula:

$$P = W/t$$

This simply means power equals work divided by time.

Let's get a better understanding of work. Work is the result of an outside force (for example, your legs straightening while standing up during the squat) moving an object (the barbell) through a distance (from the low squat position to the fully standing position). So based on this we can say that *work is force multiplied by distance.* As a formula it looks like this:

$$W = F \times d$$

Now, knowing what work is, if we go back to the first formula ($P = W/t$) and substitute force times distance ($F \times d$) for work (W), since they mean the same thing, we get another way of expressing power:

$$P = F \times d/t$$

This formula says that *power* results from *force* (you lifting the barbell) multiplied by *distance* (how far you moved the barbell) divided by *time* (how long it took you to stand up). For example, if you add more weight to the barbell and do another squat standing up (F) to the same height as before (d) and in the same amount of time as before (t), you've increased the power generated. That's because *force* was increased. Or you could keep the weight on the barbell the same as before and stand up (F) to the same height (d), only faster (t). That would also increase the power because *time* decreased. Thus, power results from the interplay of force, distance, and time.

Still with me? If so, let's see if we can simplify this even more.

You know that distance divided by time is called "velocity," which is what we more commonly call "speed." In your car you talk about speed as miles per hour. That's distance (miles) divided by (per) hours (time). So if velocity (v) is the same thing as distance divided by time (d/t), we can substitute v for d/t in the last formula, giving us an even simpler way of expressing power, especially when it comes to riding a bike:

$$P = F \times v$$

This is the final formula: *Power equals force times velocity.* It's where I wanted to take you with this somewhat roundabout way of understanding power from the perspective of physics. In bike riding, force and velocity are easier to understand than *work divided by time*, which is where we started. On a bike, force is what you put into the pedals and velocity is how fast you are turning the pedals. So now that we have the hard part out of the way, let's move on to how power is produced through the interplay of force and velocity when you ride a bike.

Power in Cycling

When you are pedaling a bicycle, force and velocity are always present and determine how much power you are creating. As you push down on the pedal, you're applying a force (F). The harder you push, the more force you are applying and therefore the greater is the power you produce. (In physics this turning force applied to the rotating pedals is called "torque." That's not too important for your understanding of power, but you may run across this word in your power meter software.)

When you are pedaling your bike, the rotating-pedal equivalent of velocity is called "revolutions per minute," or "RPM." That's a term with which you're already familiar. You may also call it "cadence." As RPM, or cadence, increases—in other words, as you pedal faster—power is potentially increasing. I said potentially because the increase depends on whether you changed gears or not. Pedaling at a higher cadence in the same gear produces more watts because pedal velocity (v) has increased.

All of this means that in order to raise your power while riding, you can either increase the force (F) you apply to the pedals or you can increase the cadence (v). In the real world of riding a bike, the way to increase the force is to shift to a higher gear and keep the cadence the same. For example, you could shift from 53×17 to 53×16 while maintaining your cadence. Force will have to increase for this to happen (you'll have to pedal harder). That will increase your power output, which in turn will increase your bike's speed. Or you could keep the force the same by not shifting gears and instead increase your cadence by turning the pedals faster—for example, by going from 85 RPM to 90 RPM. This decreases the time it takes to do the work, thus increasing power.

HOW A POWER METER WORKS

So force and cadence are what your power meter is detecting. Calculating the cadence part is easy. The meter simply measures how long it takes for the cranks to make one full revolution. Some power meters do this by having you place a magnet on a crank arm and a magnetic sensor on the frame. Others do it by electronically detecting the sine wave you produce as the cranks go around and then measuring the length of one wave to determine cadence. Force (actually, it's torque that's measured) is a bit trickier to compute.

To calculate force, your power meter has something called a "strain gauge" built in. This is the single most expensive part of a power meter and accounts for much of the price you paid for yours. It's found in the cranks, bottom bracket, rear hub, or pedals, depending on which type of power meter you have. There are generally several strain gauges in a power device to make the reading more precise. Good power meters are generally accurate to within plus or minus 2 percent.

A strain gauge is a thin, flexible strip of material with a metallic foil pattern inlaid on it. As force (torque) is increased on the pedal, the strain gauge is very slightly stretched, thus changing the shape of the metallic foil pattern. When the pattern deforms, its electrical resistance changes. The amount of this change is an indication of how much force (torque) is being applied.

So that brings us back to $P = F \times v$. Now that the power meter knows force and velocity, it can determine how much power (watts) you're creating and display that on your handlebar computer. Simple, huh?

GETTING FITTER AND FASTER WITH POWER

So if power is force times velocity ($P = F \times v$), what can you do to build more force or increase your pedaling velocity (cadence)—or both? Powerful cyclists typically do both. When necessary for performance, they can select a high gear and pedal with a high cadence. For example, a pro road cyclist who specializes in sprinting can shift to the 53-tooth chain ring and the 11-tooth cog and still turn the pedals at 105–115 RPM. This produces very high power output, often around 1,500 to 1,800 watts. That's why these cyclists sprint so fast. Most recreational riders sprint at about 600 to 1,000 watts using a much lower gear and cadence. On the endurance side, a pro triathlete in an Ironman may select a 53 ring and a 14 or16 cog with a cadence of 85–90 RPM and average around 290 watts for four and a half hours. Even though the actual numbers vary, the best athletes are capable of using both a high gear and a high cadence. More than likely you're not at such levels—yet!

Let's take a 30,000-foot view of what it will take to get there, or at least to some higher level of power than you currently are able to produce. We'll examine both force and cadence improvements. Later, in Part III, in the chapter focused on your sport, we'll take a closer look at the specifics of what you can do to train more effectively to improve power so that you become fitter and faster. There I will explain the details for merging the power of physics as explained above with the physiology of training as I've previously described it in my books *The Cyclist's Training Bible*, *The Triathlete's Training Bible*, and *The Mountain Biker's Training Bible*.

Force

For most of the athletes I've coached over the years, force is the key to greater power. They've needed more "aerobically active" muscle. These are primarily the slow-twitch, or type 1, muscle fibers you've probably read about before. Slow-twitch muscles are the ones that improve your endurance. They are not very powerful—certainly not as powerful as the type 2, or fast-twitch, muscles—yet they can contract many times before fatiguing. You have both types throughout your body, with their ratio depending mostly on genetics. Good endurance athletes have an abundance of type 1, whereas sprinters have lots of type 2. Type 2 muscles, while quite powerful, fatigue very quickly. They're great for sprinting since they can contract many times faster than type 1, but they aren't very good for endurance riding.

There are two subtypes within type 2, called "2a" and "2x." The 2a fibers have some of the same characteristics of type 1, yet they are primarily fast twitch. The 2x muscles (they used to be called "2b") have the potential to become more like 2a, meaning that their endurance qualities can be improved. With proper training, your fast-twitch muscle fibers, which are already good at producing force, can become more endurance oriented, while your slow-twitch fibers can become better at generating force. The result of all of this physiology babble is that a good training program will help you produce more force and therefore more power, as I'll describe in Part III.

Cadence

Pedaling in a very high gear with a very low cadence is not only a poor way to produce power; it is also quite inefficient. That's how those new to cycling sports usually start out. They bog down by mashing gears in the big chain ring and small cogs with a cadence of 60–70 RPM. Experienced riders, in contrast, commonly use gears that allow them to spin the cranks at a much higher cadence; 85–95 RPM is common for well-trained riders. Research has shown that such a cadence is effective and efficient for seasoned cyclists. Part III will get into the details with specific workouts to increase cadence by sport.

Basic Training

Whether you do workouts with or without a power meter, the basic training philosophy remains the same. What's changed once you start using power is the methodology: how you gauge riding intensity, design workouts, and analyze workouts and races. The common training-philosophy denominator continues to be stress.

In order to pedal with more force or a higher cadence, you must stress the body. In other words, you must do things in workouts that are slightly more challenging than what you've previously been doing. And then allow for a day or so of rest. During rest the body begins to adapt to the new level of stress, provided it wasn't excessively hard.

The changes that take place occur in the three determiners of fitness as described in exercise physiology textbooks: aerobic capacity, anaerobic threshold (AT), and economy. Let's take a quick look at each of these, as their combined changes—owing to your training—ultimately determine how fit and fast you are.

Aerobic Capacity

Also called "VO_2max," aerobic capacity is a marker of fitness that has to do with how much oxygen your body is capable of using when producing high levels of power. The more oxygen that's used when you are going at maximum intensity for several minutes, the higher is your power and the greater is your fitness. VO_2max is expressed as a number reflecting your maximum milliliters of oxygen used per kilogram of body weight per minute (ml O_2/kg/min). World-class male cyclists typically have VO_2max values above 70. The rest of us mere mortals have somewhat lower numbers. The value is about 10 percent less for women and declines as we all get older.

We look at VO_2max as one measure of endurance fitness because the energy needed to power the pedals calls for fat to be burned. Fat metabolism is based on the utilization of oxygen. When more oxygen is used at a maximal endurance workload, more fat is burned. And more power is generated. Training with a power meter will allow you to design your workouts to increase your VO_2max and also to quite precisely measure your resulting performance gains. Neither option would be feasible without a power meter.

Anaerobic Threshold

Anaerobic threshold is the point where, in a hard cycling effort, you start to close in on your limit. This point is sometimes called "lactate threshold" instead. You may also read about "ventilatory threshold" or even "OBLA" (onset of blood lactate accumulation) and "MLSS" (maximum lactate steady state). Sports scientists would be quick to point out the differences among these markers of intensity. But for our purpose here, we'll simply say that they all have to do with the submaximal intensity at which you begin to "redline" (hit the limit of your long-term, sustainable effort). At such an intensity, you experience labored breathing and realize that you won't be able to stay at this effort for long. On a rating of perceived exertion scale from 0 to 10, with 10 being maximal, you're at about a 7 when you reach your anaerobic threshold.

AT is generally expressed as a percentage of VO_2max. Riders with very good fitness have ATs around 85 percent of VO_2max. For example, a fit amateur rider with a VO_2max of 60 and AT at 82 percent would be using oxygen at the rate of 49 ml O_2/kg/min when at the anaerobic threshold. Less-fit athletes will have lower AT percentages. The closer you can get your AT to your VO_2max, the fitter you are and the faster you can ride. Although VO_2max rises only in small amounts over the course of a year for a seasoned athlete, AT can rise considerably more—if training is effective.

Again, with your power meter you'll know exactly what it takes to ride at or near AT, thus allowing you to stress and, ultimately, improve it. That simply means you'll race faster once your AT is higher. We'll come back to AT many more times in the following chapters as we discuss training with power.

Economy

You're undoubtedly familiar with this term from an understanding of the "economy" rating of your car: its miles per gallon. The more miles you can go on a gallon of gas, the more economical the car is. When you ride your bike, you also have an economy rating, only now it's meters per milliliter of oxygen. The less oxygen it takes for you to turn the pedals at any given submaximal power wattage, the more economical you are. The longer the race is, the more critical economy becomes.

For a triathlete doing an Ironman, economy is a huge determiner of performance. For a road cyclist racing a 45-minute criterium, economy is still important but not nearly as critical to the outcome. The reason for this is that the Ironman bike ride is done at a significantly lower power output than a 45-minute criterium. The crit is raced at an intensity between AT and VO_2max.

So these fitness markers are critical to such a performance. The Ironman is raced at around 70 percent of AT. During such long durations, the rider can't afford to waste energy, as the gut has a limit as to how much energy it can process from food and drink while racing. If the rate at which energy is expended owing to low economy is greater than the intake rate, the athlete will "hit the wall." The crit racer can afford to waste some energy because the race outcome will not be decided by how much energy is wasted; there is plenty of stored fuel available for such a short race, and none will need to be replaced before the race ends.

When you are riding a bike, your economy is likely between 20 and 25 percent effective, meaning that 75 to 80 percent of all the calories you burn are not producing power. Most of that lost energy is expended as radiated heat. That may seem like a lot of lost energy, but it's common. Interestingly, research reveals that athletes with high aerobic capacities tend to be somewhat less economical than athletes of otherwise similar ability with lower aerobic capacities.

Economy is dependent on many factors, several of which are outside your control, such as the length of your thighbone (long femurs relative to leg length pedal more economically than short ones) and your ratio of slow-twitch to fast-twitch muscles (slow twitch are more economical). These largely result from who your parents were.

The most significant aspect of economy over which you do have control is how you pedal. "Mashers" (riders who push big gears at low RPM) are less economical than "spinners" (riders who spin the pedals at high RPM), How rapidly you apply torque to the pedals has a significant effect on performance. With your power meter, you'll be able to determine the cadence range at which you are most economical. This is critical information for your performance.

THE BOTTOM LINE is that you've made the right decision to purchase a power meter. It is the one instrument you can buy that shows your power level and then helps you monitor your improvement in power as your training progresses. In other words, it is the best possible way to monitor and focus your training efforts. You'll be not only a more savvy rider because of it but also one who is fitter and faster than you've ever been before—if you know how to use it. That's where we will be going next.

3

Getting Started with Your Power Meter

THE PURPOSE OF THIS CHAPTER is to help you become acquainted with your power meter so that you can start using it effectively. Of course, your power meter isn't magic. You don't just mount it on your bike and all of a sudden you're training differently and become an overnight podium contender. The power meter doesn't work that way. As with any tool, you'll have to undertake some adjustment and learning to make the best use it. And there's a lot of adjusting and learning to do. Power meters are rather complex devices. You've probably started to get that sense from having read the first two chapters. And so far we've only scratched the surface.

While power meters are new as mobile devices for our bikes, they have been used as big, cumbersome clunkers in exercise physiology labs for decades. Sport scientists have used them to study performance and almost everything imaginable related to aerobic capacity, anaerobic threshold, and economy. Essentially, what you have on your bike is a powerful scientific tool. There's no doubt that it can help you become a much better rider, but you've first got to figure out how to use it.

WHAT'S ON YOUR HANDLEBARS?

Before you get serious about doing power-based workouts, I suggest you take 7 to 10 days to just ride with your new power meter. During that time, train as you normally would. If you've been using heart rate or perceived exertion to regulate the intensity of your workouts, continue to do so. That will give you time to figure out how to navigate through the power meter menu and to see in real-world fashion the relationships among power, heart rate, RPE, and speed. You'll undoubtedly learn a lot about what you are doing in workouts during this time just by observing the power display. (Again, a word of caution: Don't become so focused on the numbers that you disregard traffic and road conditions.)

After every workout, download the data to your computer and take a look at the graphs and charts. There's no need to start doing in-depth analysis now. We'll get into how to do that later. For now just become familiar with the layout, and take a look at what happens to power when you ride hard and fast, cruise along at a slow speed, climb a hill, sprint, race, or ride with a group.

After a week or so, you should be ready to make adjustments to your training based on what you see. At first, that will simply involve using the power readout on your handlebar computer to regulate workout intensity in much the same way as you may have been doing with heart rate. As you read the chapters that follow and become acquainted with the more subtle nuances of training with power, you'll be able to make other changes to how you train and race. The changes will be rather dramatic. You'll be looking at power numbers to determine how hard you are working. At first, that will take some getting used to if you've been watching heart rate or monitoring perceived exertion. Over time, the changes will gradually become smaller and more refined. Eventually, you'll be an old hand at training and racing with power. I'll help you get there one step at a time.

The first step is to understand the figures that are being displayed on your handlebar computer, which is also called a "head unit." What you see displayed there depends on the type of power meter you have. Some head units are specific to the power meters with which they came. If you have such a device, you must use the head unit that came with the meter. If there is a wire running from the power-measuring device to the head unit on your handlebars, then there's no doubt that the one that came with the device is the one you must use.

Most power meters today are wireless, and a wireless system may give you more options for head units. Many wireless systems use what's called "ANT+" technology. This is a type of wireless communication between the handlebar computer and the power-measuring device in the crank, bottom bracket, pedal, or rear hub. It's becoming a common standard. Any ANT+ power head unit can be used with any power meter that is ANT+ compatible, which allows you to choose a handlebar display and user interface without changing system types. You'll need to check the user's manual for your power meter to see what type of communication method it uses.

One of the main differences among head units is the amount of information they can show you at one time. Some have simple displays with only three data fields shown, while others show up to eight data fields all at the same time. Many head units allow you to customize the display. This is a great feature you should consider when purchasing a new head unit. Some head units are touch screens, while others rely on buttons for the interface.

Minidisplay technology has even led to a wristwatch version from Garmin, which is ANT+ compatible and displays power meter data along with run data. It's also waterproof for swimming, which makes it a good choice if you are a triathlete as all bike and run data are captured in one place.

Regardless of all these options, here are the most common items displayed by power meter head units. Not all head units use the same display abbreviations I'll use here, so you may need to consult the user guide that came with yours.

Power

This is the most basic information you need from your head unit. If you can customize the display to put the fields on your head unit wherever you want, be sure to place the current or instantaneous power display (often called "WATTS" or "PWR") in a prominent place, such as upper left, so that you can see it at a glance while riding. You'll be referring to this field more than any other.

Heart Rate

Just because you have a power meter doesn't mean you are going to forget about your heart rate. It's still quite valuable information. In Chapter 6 I'll teach you how to compare power and heart rate to accurately gauge changes in aerobic fitness. Again, if you can customize your screen display on the head unit, I'd suggest putting the "HR" readout next to power so that they can be easily seen and compared.

Duration

In addition to intensity (WATTS and HR), the other critical component of each workout is duration, or how long the ride was. This should also be displayed prominently on your head unit. You may be able to select either "TIME" or "MILES" (or perhaps "KM," for kilometers) for this field. There may even be other options, such as kiloJoules ("KJ"), that I'll explain later in this chapter. I prefer to use the TIME setting as I believe that is more valuable information when compared with power than is distance. For example, as you'll see later, intervals are usually designed based on time, not distance. And the length of time you can hold a specified power output is closely related to a given time, not a given distance. But if you want to set this field for distance and like to think in such terms about your ride duration, I won't argue with you.

Cadence

When I coach athletes who frequently use a gear I consider too high for the situation, such as climbing a hill or sprinting, and I think they could perform better in a lower gear with a higher cadence, then I recommend they set up the head unit with cadence ("RPM" or "CAD") prominently displayed. If this doesn't seem to be an issue for you, then you might want to use the next available field for other data.

Altitude

Climbing a hill is one of the major challenges of riding a bike for all athletes. Most ANT+ head units allow you to monitor climbing by setting a field to display altitude changes in feet or meters ("ALT FT" or "ALT MT"). You may even have the option to set up the grade of the climb ("% GRADE") or how much climbing you've done in a workout ("FT GAIN" or "MTR GAIN").

Some head units use the Global Positioning System (GPS) for this function, while others use barometric pressure. You may notice when standing at a stoplight that the altitude reading seems to bounce around quite a bit. That's common with both systems and reflects "handoffs" between newly arriving overhead satellites (GPS) or changes in temperature and atmospheric pressure (barometer). Which is more accurate for determining altitude, GPS or a barometer? There's a fair amount of disagreement on this matter among experts. For our purposes in riding a bike, it's not important. What we want is reliability. For example, your bathroom scale is probably not absolutely accurate to the ounce, but (you hope) it is reliable—you are confident that if it shows a change of 1 pound, what changed was you and not the scale. That's the same sort of confidence we want in your power meter.

You may even find that when you download the data after a ride, altitude changes such as feet or meters gained and starting and ending altitudes displayed on your head unit don't agree with what the software says. That's also common and has to do with the algorithms being used by each to compute altitude. Some software, such as TrainingPeaks and WKO+, correct your elevation profile based upon known coordinates in the U.S. Geological Survey (USGS) database when GPS is used. Of course, the most important piece of altitude data is feet gained rather than actual altitude at any point in the ride. Regardless, I'd recommend relying on the one shown by your software and always using it for workout analysis.

Speed

I've never met a cyclist who isn't interested in speed, so most riders set up their power meter head units to display speed in "MPH" or "KPH." In fact, however, there is a good reason to monitor speed besides the simple thrill of seeing how fast you went. In Chapter 5, I'll show you how you can use speed in conjunction with power to reliably pace steady-state races such as time trials and triathlons.

Temperature

Some head units give you the option of displaying temperature ("TEMP") in a field, while others measure it but don't display it in real time, instead opting to reveal temperature after the fact in the download to your software. Temperature measurement not only has to do with how warm and comfortable you may be on the ride but also is used to adjust the altimeter on the head unit if it relies on a barometer for altitude display. Older power meters used to be affected by big changes in temperature, but recent self-calibrating models have reduced this inaccuracy.

Other

There are a multitude of other data fields your head unit may be capable of displaying based on how it's set up and the power meter you are using. For example, it may provide such options as watts per kilogram of body weight ("W/KG"), the current power zone you are in ("ZONE"), Normalized Power™ ("NORM PWR"), Training Stress Score ("TSS"), and Intensity Factor™ ("IF"). I'll explain each of these in the following chapters. They are critical bits of data that reflect your performance. You can wait until you know more about them before deciding whether you want to display one or more of them on your head unit.

There are even more options, again depending on the power system you have. Other data fields could be dedicated to vertical ascent in meters per hour ("VAM"), kiloJoules per hour ("KJ/HR"), and left-right pedal balance ("L-R"). GPS-based head units often provide maps and directions much like those you may use when driving your car.

With all of these possibilities, setting up your handlebar display can be a daunting task. For now, you may want to keep the settings on the unit's default, just as it came out of the box. Later on, as you get the hang of what all this means, you can customize the display to better fit your needs and interests.

KILOJOULES, AVERAGE POWER, AND NORMALIZED POWER

There are several less obvious fields on your head unit that are fundamentally important for some of the workouts and analysis you'll be doing. I'll describe in later chapters how these are applied to training and racing on a bike. If you are a bit confused by any of these or other terms when you encounter them in this book, on your head unit, or in software, you can refer to the Glossary for help.

KiloJoules

In Chapter 2, I told you that watts (the unit of measure for power) is an indicator of how much energy you're expending during a ride. That may have seemed a strange way to explain something that deals with how much force you are generating and how fast your cadence is. But they are really one and the same. The greater your power is owing to the combination of force and cadence, the more energy it takes to pedal the bike.

As humans we usually think of energy expended in Calories. A Calorie (with a capital "C") is the same as 1,000 calories, and the scientific term for the Calories we burn is "kiloCalories." The distinction is pointless in general conversation, but it is useful for training. You see, mechanical energy, the kind you create on your bike and that your power device senses, is expressed in "kiloJoules." This is what your power meter is measuring and what shows up on the head unit. And the relationship between kiloCalories and kiloJoules gives you a good picture of how much fuel you burn, which in turn can help you plan your nutrition.

Here's how it works: 1 kiloCalorie equals about 4 kiloJoules (actually, it's 4.184, but we don't need to be nearly that precise here). Humans pedaling a bike are roughly 25 percent efficient—and that's probably a bit high but okay for our purpose. This means that only about one-fourth of the biological energy you generate (kiloCalories) during a ride is converted into the mechanical energy that drives the bike (kiloJoules). The rest is mostly lost to the heat your body gives off, no matter whether it's a hot or a cold day. So if you are 25 percent efficient in terms of mechanical energy generated, and 1 kiloCalorie is about 4 kiloJoules, then only about 1 kiloJoule is actually realized as mechanical energy for every 1 kiloCalorie of biological energy burned. What all of this means is that when your head unit shows 500 kiloJoules at the end of a ride, you have used about 500 kiloCalories. That may be around 10 percent higher than the actual number, but individual riders vary so much that this number is close enough for training purposes. And it's very useful, as we'll see later on.

Average Power

If you've been using a speedometer or heart rate monitor when riding, you're used to dealing with average speed and average heart rate. Average power is a similar metric: It is the total of all the watts generated during a ride divided by the number of time units (for example, minutes) during which the data was collected. This calculation is always going on within the head unit and can be displayed during the ride or afterward in your software download. Average power is quite simple—so simple that it is not always the most useful measurement for our purposes. Instead, as you'll see in a moment, you will want to use Normalized Power (NP) for most of your analysis.

Normalized Power: Why Not Just Average Power?

Even though I will occasionally use average power as a metric in the chapters that follow, I'll frequently refer to Normalized Power as it is better at taking into account what you experience while riding. Normalized Power is simply an expression of average power adjusted for the range of variability during a ride and therefore more closely reflects the effort or metabolic cost of a ride than does average power. So what does "normalized" mean?

One way to normalize data is to divide one set by another. For example, we could normalize the power of several riders for their weights (and, in fact, we will do so in a later chapter). To do this, we divide power by body weight. For example, if rider A weighs 180 pounds and his average power for a given ride was 210 watts, his power normalized for weight would be 1.17 watts per pound (210 ÷ 180 = 1.17). We could compare that with rider B's data on the same course. If B weighs 120 pounds and had an average power of 150 watts, her power normalized for weight would be 1.25 (150 ÷ 120 = 1.25). So we could conclude that even though A puts out far more average power than B, B is actually more powerful pound for pound. That relationship becomes very important under some circumstances, such as climbing a hill, which we'll get to later. But for now, that's what is meant by *normalizing*.

NP compares the range of variability of power during a ride with the average power of the ride. So when you see the word "normalized," you are being tipped off that we have altered the parameters to be examined. Let's see if we can get a better grip on this concept.

If you've had a chance to download and look at one of your power charts from a ride, you certainly will have noticed that there are lots of spikes in the chart. If you compare the power chart with the heart rate chart for the same ride, you'll see that heart rate doesn't spike nearly as much. That's because power generation is quite variable and the power meter is very sensitive to change, whereas heart rate doesn't change much at all. If you were a machine, we could design you to create steady, even power. But you aren't a machine; you're human, and humans expend energy with lots of high and low spikes. Every time there is a rising spike in power, you are expending more energy than if you rode with perfect steadiness and no spike at all. Average power doesn't account for these minute changes in power and therefore in the energy you used to pedal. Normalized Power does.

The concept of Normalized Power is critical for power meter training because it reveals the true effort of a ride by accounting for variability. I will refer to NP frequently throughout the following chapters; to help lock it in, let me give you a real-life example of NP from two of my recent rides.

Not too long ago, I had only 1 hour to work out between other commitments. You know how it is sometimes—you have to shoehorn bike rides in whenever you can by working around other responsibilities. I happen to live at the top of a 1-mile hill that is about a 5 percent grade. What I did for this short workout was repeats on the hill for 1 hour. On the climbs I rode at a hard effort with several short surges thrown in all the way to the top. Once at the crest, I turned around and coasted back down without pedaling. After 1 hour my average power was 141 watts. The next day I was a bit tired from the hard workout the day before, so I went for a moderate-effort, steady ride on a flat course. Interestingly, my average power was once again 141 watts. Now, there was nothing about those two workouts that was even remotely the same except for the average power. I burned a lot more calories per hour climbing and descending the hill than I did riding steadily. In fact, NP reflected this difference. The hill-climbing workout had an NP of 176 watts. For the moderate-effort ride, it was 149 watts. If I had only the average powers to compare, I would assume the effort and the metabolic cost were the same for both rides. They obviously weren't, and NP revealed this.

So what NP is actually telling us is what the workout *felt* like, which is a much more revealing training component than a simple measurement of average power level for the ride. In my example, the hill repeats felt much harder than the steady, moderate-effort ride, and NP reflected a difference that average power would not. Normalized Power also gives us a much better idea of the energy cost of a ride. Doing surges on the hill burned a lot more calories than riding steadily. That's why we will use NP for much of our riding and analysis. (If you are still unsure about what Normalized Power means, please take a few minutes to reread this section.)

POWER'S RELATIONSHIPS WITH TIME AND HEART RATE

Earlier I suggested that in setting up your head unit, you should place duration and heart rate in prominent fields near current or instantaneous power since they are the next most important data fields. After riding with your new power meter for a week or so, you may notice some interesting things happening in the relationships between power and time and power and heart rate. These are critical relationships for training and racing, which we'll explore in much greater detail later in the book. For now, let's look at how they interact.

Power and Time

You're probably already starting to get some thoughts about how to train with power. From the last section, you should now understand that the power data on your handlebars is closely related to your effort and expended energy while riding a bike. Power is also closely related to the duration—time—of the workout or race or a segment of one of those.

As time increases, power decreases if you are working at or near maximal effort. This should be obvious by now if you've gotten in a few rides with your power meter. You've probably done a short sprint of a few seconds at some point in a workout or race and seen the spike in power on your head unit and in the software chart after downloading the session. Do you think you could hold that same sprint power output for an hour? Absolutely not. Would you be able to hold that sprint power for a minute? Again, absolutely not if the sprint was an all-out effort of only a few seconds.

Your personal power levels are specific to the duration of the output. As the time of the workout increases, the normalized and average powers will decrease if you are riding with a high effort. This should be obvious in racing. It is also true of intervals, which we'll examine in much greater detail in later chapters. Power and time are inversely related—when one changes, the other changes in the opposite direction. The "5 Percent Rule" explains this.

The 5 Percent Rule says that when the duration of a session (or a segment) doubles, the power you generate to ride at a maximal effort for the longer duration decreases by about 5 percent. For example, if you do a short time trial race that takes 20 minutes and you will soon do another that is expected to take 40 minutes, you can estimate that the power of the longer one will be about 5 percent less than that of the shorter race. So if your average power was 240 watts in the 20-minute race, the estimated average power for the 40-minute race would be 228 watts ($240 \times 0.05 = 12$; $240 - 12 = 228$). The 5 Percent Rule is helpful whenever you try to calculate from a known duration to a new duration so that you can estimate the required power for a maximal effort. (There is an interesting exception to this rule that I'll explain in Chapter 4 in the section that describes how to determine your Functional Threshold Power.)

Power and Heart Rate

You've probably been training with a heart rate monitor for a long time now. They've been around since the late 1970s and can be found on nearly all riders at the start lines of races. To make the best use of your heart rate monitor, you've set up zones. In the next chapter, I'll show you how to set power zones to use in much the same way as you've done with your heart rate zones. But before doing that, I want to make sure you understand the relationship between these two sets of zones as it is confusing for many athletes, especially when they start comparing heart rate zones and power zones during rides.

In your first year or so of serious training, your heart rate zones stabilize as you become more aerobically fit. Once your zones have stabilized, there will be only slight changes found in testing over the course of a season. These changes are more likely the result of how tired or rested you are when testing; they could also be due to factors such as diet, air temperature, and even motivation, rather than how fit you are. Heart rate zones are quite constant. They change very little.

In contrast, power zones may vary a lot during a season. And that's a good thing. As your endurance fitness improves, you are capable of achieving greater power outputs at any given heart rate. (In Chapter 7, I'll show you how to use this change to measure aerobic fitness improvement.) This means your power zones will change significantly as your fitness changes— yet your heart rate zones will remain unchanged. The two sets of zones may be about the same early in the season when fitness is at a low point. In other words, in the early base period when you are riding in heart rate zone 2, you may also be in power zone 2, although they still won't match exactly. But in the build period, shortly before your first targeted race, you may be in heart rate zone 2 but power zone 3. Don't be freaked out by this. It's a good thing and will help you understand why to gauge intensity, we will use power zones, rather than heart rate, in most of your training.

MAKING SENSE OF IT ALL

One of the great benefits of training with power comes from examining the graphs after the workout is over. In doing this, you can see if you are achieving the markers of race readiness you've set for yourself. You will be able to answer the questions "Am I becoming more fit?" and "What should I do next in my training?" This is analysis. It can be a very simple process involving a brief glance at certain graphs, or it can be highly complex activity with nearly as much time spent analyzing the data as it took to create it on a ride. If you do no analysis at all, then there is little reason to have a power meter. In that case, it's just an expensive accessory on your handlebars.

Do You Need Power Software?

The answer to that question is "yes." You definitely need software to make your power meter a complete tool for better athletic performance. In the remainder of this book, I'll show you how to quickly view your workout data so that you can see how you're doing. It's not hard or confusing or complicated. Anyone can do it who knows what to look for and how to use a computer. Viewing your data also doesn't have to take a lot of time. A five-minute look at a few key reports after each ride, or even every few days, will reveal all you need to know.

The greater question has to do with what software you should use. Appendix C lists all the power software available as of this writing. Your power meter probably came with analysis software; you may have already loaded it and taken a look at some of your workouts. I'm sure the data looks confusing. But don't give up. It will all begin to make sense over time. This book will help.

Understand that not all software shows everything I'll explain in later chapters. And some charts on your software won't be covered here. All of the metrics described in this book are found in the TrainingPeaks and WKO+ software (both available at TrainingPeaks.com). If you want to use software that shows exactly what is covered here, then these are good options. TrainingPeaks is an online software service, so all of your data is stored on its servers. You must have Internet access to use the service, but it's available from any computer. WKO+ is a desktop application, and the data is stored on your computer's hard drive. With WKO+ you may also upload it to TrainingPeaks for backup in case something goes wrong with your computer. WKO+ is compatible only with PCs; it can't be used with a Mac unless you have virtualization software that enables Windows software to run on a Mac.

What About a Coach?

Some riders strongly dislike anything to do with analysis. They want to know how they are training and what they can do to get fitter and faster, but they don't want to even glance at software charts and graphs. My wife is one such person—a strong rider who has no interest in analysis. She has me to help (I hope that's not the only reason she keeps me around!). If you'd like help, I highly recommend hiring a coach to do your analysis and planning. I've trained hundreds of cycling, triathlon, and mountain bike coaches to use the methods explained here. You can find them listed at cycleops.com/coaches.

HAVING READ PART I, you now should have a basic understanding of what a power meter is and generally how it can help you become a stronger cyclist. Now it's time to move on to Part II and how you can start training and racing with your power meter to become fitter and faster.

PART II

HOW CAN I TRAIN MORE EFFECTIVELY USING MY POWER METER?

4

Your Power Zones

BY NOW YOU SHOULD HAVE a good understanding of how your power meter works and what it can do for you. In this and the following chapters, we will get into how you can use your power meter to produce greater fitness. By the end of this chapter, you will have your power-training zones set up and know the basics of how to use those zones for workouts and races.

POWER ZONES

Power zones are a simple training tool: They are the various power intensities that you use to plan and execute your training. If you have used a heart rate monitor, you are familiar with the process of setting up your heart rate zones for your training. Power zones are similar, and we use seven of them: Active Recovery (zone 1), Aerobic Endurance (zone 2), Tempo (zone 3), Lactate Threshold (zone 4), VO_2max (zone 5), Anaerobic Capacity (zone 6), and Sprint Power (zone 7). The primary difference between heart rate zones and power zones is that with power, we set each of the seven zones as a percentage of your Functional Threshold Power (FTP) instead of a percentage of a reference heart rate. But what on earth is Functional Threshold Power? Glad you asked; read on for the answer to the surest way yet to build your cycling fitness.

FTP—YOUR MOST IMPORTANT NUMBER

The first time you set up your heart rate zones, you had two ways of doing it. In the early days of using a heart rate monitor, you may have used your "maximum heart rate" (MHR) to do this. Knowing that number, you'd then use percentages of MHR to assign zones. In recent years, there has been a shift toward basing heart rate zones on percentages of one's "lactate threshold" heart rate, which you also may have heard called "anaerobic threshold" heart rate. The latter is a much more precise way of establishing zones, as it's based on the point at which you begin to redline. This critical piece of information is unique to you and has a lot more application to high-performance racing than does MHR.

Two athletes with the same MHR won't necessarily have the same "lactate threshold heart rate" (LTHR). That presents a problem. If they have the same zones based on MHR, when they are working out, they will not experience the same sensations of effort. The one with the lower LTHR will be forced to work harder than the higher-LTHR athlete. The one with the lower LTHR needs to have lower zones despite his or her MHR. For this reason, setting up zones based on LTHR is now becoming the norm.

The challenge of basing zones on lactate or anaerobic threshold (also sometimes referred to as ventilatory threshold, onset of blood lactate accumulation, or maximum lactate steady state) is the sciencespeak confusion factor. The terminology simply isn't user-friendly or clear for nonscientists. Few athletes know what all of these terms mean, so they feel compelled to go to a lab or clinic to be tested in order to simply set zones. Then once they have the lab-test data, they sometimes discover that there are different definitions in science of what lactate threshold means. And so the data often turns out to be useless. Money wasted and still no zones.

In the sections that follow, I'll explain a relatively new way of setting power zones that doesn't require an understanding of physiology or an expensive visit to a lab or clinic. It's a simple concept called "Functional Threshold Power." We'll look at a couple of ways you can determine your FTP, and then we'll set your power zones as a percentage of your FTP.

What Is FTP?

Functional Threshold Power is the brainchild of a sports scientist and road cyclist by the name of Andrew Coggan, PhD. He came up with the idea in the early 2000s. Dr. Coggan's way of setting power zones is so simple it's elegant. It is based on the notion that a fit athlete can maintain his or her lactate threshold intensity for about an hour. So rather than an athlete going to a lab or clinic to directly determine lactate threshold power, he came up with the idea of finding it by discovering the power that athlete can hold for 60 minutes. Brilliant!

Besides the simplicity, what I like about this method is that it eliminates all of the scientific mumbo jumbo about lactate and the out-of-pocket cost associated with doing a lab or clinic test. It's also a real-world solution, meaning that it directly translates to the reality of racing out on the road. Races are not conducted in labs or clinics on stationary ergometers. Dr. Coggan's concept avoids all that in favor of a measurement taken from the roads you already ride.

Determining Your FTP

Dr. Coggan's method for determining your FTP is not perfect. The major problem is the need to do a 60-minute test. Such a field test would certainly challenge your capacity for suffering. It takes great focus and motivation for anyone to go out on the road or get on an indoor trainer (an off-road trail would not be suitable for the test) and ride a solo workout as hard as possible for 60 minutes. Fortunately, there are other ways of finding your FTP that don't require such a long, agonizing sufferfest. Here are some of the more common alternatives, from the most reliable to the least.

Races. Do you have a local bicycle time trial that's available, especially one that would take you about an hour to complete? Your average power for such an event would be precisely what you need for calculating FTP. A 40-km time trial would be about right for many athletes. The 40-km leg of a triathlon or duathlon would not, however, as in those events you have to hold back on the bike in order to run well. That would skew the results and make the numbers a bit too low.

Almost as good as a time trial is a 1-hour criterium for road cyclists. Even though it's not steady, a rider's NP for such a race is usually quite close to FTP if the race is a hard one. But if the field sits up and lets the break ride away, then the results are unlikely to accurately predict FTP. You need a solid hour of hard racing to make the measurement useful. This is when Normalized Power really shines in comparison with average power as it takes into account the positive and negative spikes in power production common for such races. For a well-paced time trial (more on pacing shortly), the difference between Normalized Power and average power will be inconsequential.

The race you use could even be a time trial or criterium that lasts less than 1 hour. But let's stop and consider an important point here before getting into the details. Whenever we have a test duration that isn't 1 hour, we are in the realm of *estimating* rather than *measuring* FTP. That opens the door for error. And the further the test is from 1 hour, the greater is the potential for error. So bear in mind that what I'm going to explain from here on in this entire section isn't as accurate as doing a 1-hour race as a test. But you probably won't be off by much if we keep the difference to 30 minutes or less.

Let's say you are going to use a shorter race for estimating FTP. In this case, you'd apply the 5 Percent Rule described in Chapter 3. To refresh your memory, the 5 Percent Rule says that when the duration of a maximal effort is doubled, the power decreases by about 5 percent. This means that if you did a time trial or criterium race that took about 30 minutes, you would subtract 5 percent to estimate FTP.

For example, let's say you did a 20-km time trial in 30 minutes and your average power was 260 watts. By subtracting 5 percent (13 watts), you would estimate that your FTP is 247 watts (260 – 13 = 247). Even if your time was a few minutes more or less than 30 minutes, perhaps between 25 and 35 minutes, we could draw the same conclusion since it's only an estimate anyway. What you should be doing is closely monitoring several different methods of estimating FTP and drawing conclusions from all of them in order to make your FTP more precise.

30-minute test. Although a 1-hour race is the best way to determine FTP, you can do a field test instead, and one that is shorter than 60 minutes. This is the most common method I use with the athletes whom I coach and with whom I consult. It's simple. Warm up, then ride on the road (not a trail, if you're a mountain biker) or an indoor trainer for 30 minutes as hard as you can. (Note: Most riders find that doing this test on an indoor trainer is much more difficult.) Your average power is a good estimate of your FTP *without your even subtracting the 5 percent described above.* I'll explain this because it seems contrary to what I said earlier.

When you do a race, you will always push yourself harder than in a workout. In workouts there's nothing on the line. There are no awards, no podiums, and no pats on the back. So we just don't work as hard as we are capable of doing in a race. We are much more likely to feel a bit sorry for ourselves in a workout and so back off—but only slightly. How much easier do we ride? About 5 percent. How cool is that? We've canceled out the 5 Percent Rule by doing the 30 minutes as a workout instead of a race. That means a 30-minute solo test is about the same as a 60-minute race when it comes to your average power. But notice that I said *solo.* You can't do a 30-minute field test with a training partner or in a group. That changes everything. In that case you'd need to subtract 5 percent.

Pacing this test is the challenge, especially the first few times you do it. The more times you do the 30-minute FTP-determination test, the better you'll get at pacing. At first, however, you're likely to start too fast and then fade as the test progresses. That's likely to produce an average power that's inaccurate. Here's how to pace the test. Start with what you believe or know your FTP to have been from a recent race, test, or other method as described below (including estimation based on weight and personal modifiers). Hold this power for the first 10 minutes of the test. At that point, decide if the power you are maintaining is too hard or too easy, and then make an adjustment up or down accordingly. Repeat this self-assessment of power every 5 minutes thereafter until you are done. Your average power for the entire 30 minutes will be a good estimation of your FTP.

To help the accuracy of this method, you must keep conditions similar from test to test. That includes such variables as riding on the road or an indoor trainer, the course you use, the time of day for the test, warm-up, equipment (including tire pressure), weather conditions, rest status, and pre-ride food and drink. There will likely be some conditions that change from one test to the next. The most likely is weather. But control as many as you can for the sake of accuracy.

Workouts. While riding, pay attention to your perceived exertion, especially when doing steady efforts for several minutes, as when climbing a hill. Whenever you sense that your exertion level is steady at about 7 on a 0 (low) to 10 (high) scale, look at your current wattage. It's likely close to your FTP. You could also use your software graph of the ride to find these segments after the workout. These are estimations that should help you to narrow down the range in which your FTP is likely to be found.

Heart rate. Don't use your heart rate zones to set your power zones. For example, when riding in heart rate zone 2, you are not necessarily going to be in power zone 2. You may recall from Chapter 3 that this is because heart rate zones stay relatively stable, while power zones change significantly relative to fitness changes. Although the two zones may overlap quite a bit early in the training season when fitness is low, the overlap will decrease as your fitness increases. The only heart rate and power numbers that may be the same, or at least close, are your LTHR and FTP. When riding steadily for several minutes at LTHR, you should be about at your FTP, so that is one simple way of estimating it.

Here is a simple way of testing for an estimated FTP based on LTHR. On an indoor bicycle trainer, warm up for 10 to 20 minutes. Then start a graded-exercise test consisting of several 4-minute stages separated by 1-minute recoveries. The first stage begins at a power that is roughly 80 watts below what you currently think your FTP is based on race data, previous testing, or a rough estimation as suggested below. Each subsequent work stage is increased by 10 watts. You'll have to watch the head unit closely, being sure to stay at the prescribed wattage for each stage. Pedal for 4 minutes at a comfortable cadence in whatever gear allows you to create this power output; observe the response of your heart rate. It will gradually increase in the first minute or two and then stabilize for the remainder. At the end of each 4-minute stage, pedal at a very easy effort for 1 minute. Then start the next stage. This continues until the stage in which LTHR is observed. Be sure to finish that 4-minute stage. The average power for this last stage should be close to your FTP.

Estimation. This could be the least accurate way of coming up with your FTP, but I've found it to be remarkably close for many riders. This is an estimation based primarily on body weight and other personal factors. It involves some math, so you're likely to need a calculator. There are five steps in estimating your FTP this way, some of which may not apply to you.

Step 1. Double your body weight in pounds. This is your base number. Example: A body weight of 150 pounds means a base of 300 (150 × 2 = 300).

Step 2. If you are a woman, subtract 10 percent from the base number found in step 1. Example: A 120-pound woman's base is 216 (120 × 2 = 240; 240 − 24 = 216).

Step 3. Subtract from your base number half a percentage point (0.5 percent) for every year beyond age 35. Example: If the 150-pound rider in step 1 is 50 years old, he would subtract 7.5 percent from 300 (50 − 35 = 15;

15 × 0.005 = 0.075). This would modify the base number to 277 (300 × 0.075 = 22.5; 300 − 22.5 = 277.5).

Step 4. If you live at about 5,000 feet altitude, subtract an additional 5 percent. For every additional 1,000 feet of altitude above 5,000, subtract another 1 percent. Example: For a 35-year-old rider with a base of 277 who lives at an altitude of about 5,000 feet, the adjusted base would be 263 (277 × 0.05 = 13.85; 277 − 13.85 = 263.15). If you are in the first month of adapting to a higher altitude, then double the percentage subtracted. Note that short visits to high altitude require an adjustment of your FTP.

Step 5. If you ride your bike fewer than six times a week, you will need to make one more adjustment. This is likely to affect triathletes more than road cyclists or mountain bikers. The less frequently you ride, the lower your FTP is likely to be. So if you typically ride five times a week, subtract 2 percent. If you ride four times weekly, subtract 4 percent. If you usually ride three times in a week, subtract 7 percent. For two rides weekly, subtract 10 percent. Example: A rider with a base of 277 who rides three times each week would have an adjusted base of 258 (277 × 0.07 = 19.39; 277 − 19.39 = 257.61).

Your final number is an estimation of your FTP. Remember, though, that it could be well off the mark. It's a rough estimate at best, particularly because there are variables besides body weight, gender, age, altitude, and training frequency that could also affect your FTP. For example, the type of weight you have would influence your estimated FTP. Excess fat or muscle, especially upper-body muscle, will skew the results. If you have a considerable amount of either of these, then your estimated FTP from the above steps is likely too high. Knowing lean body mass from body composition measurement is a better predictor if fat is an issue. That won't help overly muscular riders, however. Then there is also the weight of your bike. This is not included in the steps above, but it certainly is an issue. A heavy bike will lower an otherwise high FTP just as excess body weight does. Bike weight is especially significant for a small woman. An 18-pound bike is a heavy load to carry uphill for a 100-pound rider. In short, I wouldn't suggest relying on estimation beyond just getting started. At the first opportunity, use a more accurate measure from the above possibilities.

Keeping FTP Current

Over the course of the season, you may do some mix of the above methods for estimating FTP. You are likely to use all of them, some more than others. The one I use the most for the athletes I work with is the 30-minute test. What's most important is that you keep your FTP current. Check it at least every 6 weeks and preferably more frequently. It's a good idea to schedule testing or racing in your annual training plan with this in mind. Testing should be done after a few days of rest.

You could also simply pay close attention to changes in how hard a given power output feels in workouts and races. You may find, for example, that after three or four weeks of repeating a given workout, the effort seems easier. This is a good sign that your FTP has increased—along with your fitness—so this is the time to measure it.

FTP is the most easily measured and accurate way of determining changes in fitness. Your most important training objective during the season is to raise your FTP to as high a level as possible. Why? Let's look at it this way: If your closest competitor has exactly the same VO_2max as you, the rider who prevails on race day will be the one with the higher FTP. In fact, a high FTP can make up for a relatively low VO_2max. So if your FTP is higher, you can perform well even if others have genetics on their side. Pure and simple, training is largely about FTP.

YOUR PERSONAL POWER ZONES

In this section, we will set up your power zones based on FTP. If you haven't been able to do any testing or a race, then simply use an estimate as described above. If you already know your FTP, then you're ready to go.

Training with power zones is much like training with heart rate zones—only better. Heart rate is slow to respond to increases in intensity. Your power meter will show change almost immediately. This is important when you are doing intervals, and the shorter the intervals, the more important this becomes. At the start of an interval, if you are relying on heart rate to gauge intensity, there may be a 2-minute wait as your heart begins to beat faster. During this time, you are forced to guess how hard to work. Most athletes guess too high and find they have to slow down when heart rate finally catches up. Others decide that the interval doesn't even start until heart rate reaches the prescribed level. So a 3-minute interval becomes 5 minutes. None of this happens with a power meter. Within three pedal strokes, you know if you are at the level you wanted.

Once your power zones are set, you're ready to start training—and reaping the benefits of having a power meter.

How to Set Your Power Zones

Just as you have probably done with heart rate zones, you'll set power zones using fixed percentages. For power zones, they are based on your FTP. If you know your FTP, use Table 4.1 to determine your zones using the percentages in the "% of FTP" column. The "RPE" column relates power zones to a rating of perceived exertion scale of 0 (low) to 10 (high) plus "maximal." The "Description" column describes what to expect from each zone as far as sensations of fatigue, workout type, and most common race categories.

Zone 3

I have already offered the opinion that your most important training objective during the season is to raise your FTP to as high a level as possible. I have found it to be the best marker of changes in fitness short of going to an exercise physiology lab for extensive—and expensive—testing throughout the season. It works.

If your most important training objective is to raise FTP, how do you go about doing so? Put another way, what zone is best for raising FTP?

As far as improving FTP, the greatest return on investment comes from riding in zone 4, especially at or around FTP. However, the "cost"—mental stress, time to recover, and risk of injury—of training frequently at such high intensity is too great for most riders. It's so great, in fact, that riders generally need two or more days of recovery after such a training session before zone 4 training can be repeated. With less recovery time between zone 4 interval sessions, fatigue accumulates rapidly and motivation wanes.

So while it's generally a good idea to do some zone 4 training, especially in preparation for an event in which zone 4 is race effort, a steady regimen of FTP-intensity workouts is not recommended. Instead, I frequently use zone 3 in training athletes. I have found this to be quite effective in producing FTP gains. Zone 3 workouts can be done much more frequently and with longer workout durations than zone 4 sessions. The risk associated with such workouts is also low.

TABLE 4.1 # POWER-BASED TRAINING ZONES

ZONE	NAME	% OF FTP	RPE	DESCRIPTION
1	ACTIVE RECOVERY	<55	<2	Often referred to as "easy spinning" or "light pedal pressure," this is a very low level of exercise. Minimal sensation of effort or fatigue. Continual conversation possible. Typically used for active recovery after hard workouts or races, between intervals, and for socializing.
2	AEROBIC ENDURANCE	56–75	2–3	Classic "long, slow distance" training. Intensity most age-group athletes will use in an Ironman triathlon. Effort and fatigue generally low but increase during prolonged, steady riding at this intensity. Concentration generally required to maintain this effort only at the high end of the range and during longer rides. Continual conversation possible. Frequent training sessions of around 90 minutes to 2 hours or less in this zone generally well tolerated. Complete recovery from longer workouts often takes more than 24 hours.
3	TEMPO	76–90	4–5	Typical intensity of brisk group rides, sitting in on a fast road race peloton, elite Ironman triathlon, most age-group half-Ironman triathlons, and mountain bike marathon events. Long, steady rides of 20 to 60 minutes. Significantly greater sensation of effort and fatigue than in zone 2. Breathing deeper and more rhythmic than in zone 2. Conversation somewhat broken. Recovery from zone 3 training sessions takes longer than after zone 2 workouts. Consecutive days of zone 3 training possible if duration not excessive.
4	LACTATE THRESHOLD	91–105	6–7	This zone includes FTP. Commonly used in time trials and triathlon bike legs of about 30- to 90-minute durations. Sensations of effort and fatigue high. Breathing labored, conversation difficult. Mentally challenging. Interval training at this intensity is common, with relatively long durations of 6 to 20 minutes and recoveries about one-fourth as long. Consecutive days of training in zone 4 possible but not common. Zone 4 training requires focused recovery.
5	VO$_2$max	106–120	7–8	Typical intensity of surges in a bike race. Other than in draft-legal events or when climbing short hills at sprint and Olympic distances, triathletes seldom race at this intensity. Interval training is the most common use of this intensity, with repeats and recoveries of about 2 to 6 minutes. Effort and fatigue very high. More than 20 to 30 minutes of total training time in a workout difficult. Conversation not possible. Recovery critical. Consecutive days of zone 5 training extremely difficult and seldom recommended.
6	ANAEROBIC CAPACITY	121–150	>8	Short episodes at this intensity are common in criteriums and in road and mountain bike races but are highly unusual in triathlon. Training involves short (30 seconds to 2 minutes), high-intensity intervals to increase anaerobic capacity. Effort and fatigue extremely high, and conversation not possible. Consecutive days of zone 6 training not recommended.
7	SPRINT POWER	>150	Maximal	This zone is used for very short, very high-intensity efforts, such as standing starts on the track and short sprints of less than 30 seconds' duration in road races. This zone generally places greater stress on muscles than on energy-production systems.

SOURCE: Adapted from http://freewebs.com/velodynamics2/traininglevels.pdf with permission of the author, Andrew Coggan, PhD.

This flies in the face of the commonly offered training advice of avoiding moderate-effort workouts. Don't let that bother you. I used to think that way until I tried these workouts. I learned that zone 3, especially the upper range, is quite effective for improving FTP. You'll see it used extensively in the next section and in the Appendix A workouts. There is no reason to avoid zone 3. You should use it frequently, especially in the base period when general fitness is the focus and in the build period for maintenance of FTP while race-specific fitness is being developed.

Workouts and Power Zones

In order to increase your FTP, the primary focus of your training should be on producing *aerobically active muscle*. That is, you want to pursue training that improves your muscles' oxygen-using capabilities. Muscle, not your heart, must be the focus of your training if you are to raise your FTP. Physiologically speaking, the aerobic adaptations we are seeking in and around the muscles that power the bike include increasing these factors:

- The muscles' ability to process lactate
- Blood plasma volume
- Aerobic enzymes
- Muscle glycogen storage
- The size of slow-twitch muscle fibers
- Muscle capillary density
- The conversion of muscle fibers from type 2x to type 2a

How should you train to accomplish all of this in order to improve your aerobically active muscle? This brings us to the topic of workouts—the most basic element of training.

For the sake of simplicity, I divide all workouts into six categories called "abilities." All of the workouts in a given ability have similar intensities, meaning their power requirements are about the same. Here are the six abilities with workout examples for each. (You can find more in-depth descriptions for these abilities in some of my other books: *The Cyclist's Training Bible, The Triathlete's Training Bible,* and *The Mountain Biker's Training Bible.*) Chapters 7 through 10 will explain the sport-specific nuances of each ability and how they are arranged, or "periodized," throughout the season. Here I only want to introduce the concept of abilities and show their relationships to the above power zones. You will see more detailed examples of these workouts in Appendix A.

Aerobic endurance. For the cyclist and triathlete, this is the most basic of the six abilities. It is critical for success in all endurance sports. Aerobic endurance workouts are quite effective for initiating most of the muscles' physiological adaptations listed above. These workouts employ extended, steady rides in zone 2 and in the lower range of zone 3.

Muscular force. This is also a basic ability. The purpose here is to improve the muscles' ability to apply force to the pedals. Recall from Chapter 2 that power is the result of force times velocity ($P = F \times v$). Muscular force can be increased with very brief, maximal-effort repeats in zone 7 using a high gear (F) and a very low cadence (v). A common workout is 8 to 12 revolutions of the pedals from a standing start while staying seated using a high gear such as 53×14. These are commonly done on a hill to increase the force required.

Muscular force intervals are quite stressful not only for the muscles but also for the joints, especially the knees. You must pay attention to unusual leg sensations and be prepared to stop this workout if something simply doesn't feel right. Long recoveries in zone 1, on the order of 3 to 5 minutes, are common between these intense repetitions as full recovery of the muscle is needed to produce high intensity and the desired results. Short recoveries and fatigue will diminish the benefits.

Speed skills. This is the last of the basic abilities and is closely related to the v in $P = F \times v$, and also to your efficiency. A common difference between novice and advanced athletes is how smoothly the latter pedal. Applying force to the pedals at high cadence in a rhythmic and effortless manner is critical for success over long distances and takes years of training to master. I've never known a high-level cyclist who mashes with a low cadence or who pedals sloppily. The ability to spin smoothly is a common characteristic of the best riders.

Speed skills workouts typically involve pedaling drills such as isolated leg training and high-cadence spinning. These drills may be included within workouts that have a primary focus on any of the other abilities, such as during the warm-up or cooldown.

Power output is not a good measure of speed skills improvement. Over the course of several weeks early in the season, if you have been a masher, you should gradually be able to increase your cadence in higher gears. This is the result of combining muscular force and speed skills training (again, $P = F \times v$). A higher cadence in any given gear, of course, means greater power.

Muscular endurance. This is an advanced ability as it is closely tied to race performance in all endurance events. The purpose of such training is to improve most of the physiological adaptations listed above but especially the first: the muscles' ability to process lactate.

Contrary to what you may be thinking, lactate—usually referred to as "lactic acid"—is not a cause of fatigue, nor does it cause muscle soreness. Those are myths that refuse to go away. Lactate is produced by the muscle cells during exercise, and it is actually reused by the muscles to produce energy so that you can keep on pedaling hard. The burning sensation you experience as a harbinger of impending fatigue is caused by hydrogen ions released into the body's fluids, including blood, as lactate seeps out of the muscle during a hard effort. Muscular endurance workouts will improve your muscles' ability to reprocess the lactate to create more energy and quickly remove the hydrogen ions.

Muscular endurance workouts are done in the upper end of zone 3 and in zone 4. The differences between zone 3 aerobic endurance workouts and zone 3 muscular endurance workouts are the zone range, duration, and volume of the intensity within a workout. Muscular endurance involves working at the upper end of zone 3 with longer durations and greater zone volume within the session than in aerobic endurance training. And, as mentioned, muscular endurance includes zone 4 workout intensity.

A common muscular endurance workout is 4 intervals of 20 minutes each at the upper end of zone 3 with 5-minute recoveries in zone 1. Another is 5 repeats of 6 minutes each in zone 4 with 90-second zone 1 recoveries between them. Muscular endurance intervals may be done on hills or on flat terrain.

Anaerobic endurance. These advanced-ability workouts are quite common for road cyclists and mountain bikers as racing in these sports frequently requires anaerobic efforts beyond FTP. Triathletes are less likely to do anaerobic endurance training other than to improve VO_2max. Workouts for this ability are done in zones 5 and 6. A typical session is 5 intervals of 3 minutes' duration done at zone 5 with 3-minute recoveries in zone 1. Another is 3 sets of 5 repeats of 30 seconds' duration done in zone 6 with 30-second recoveries in zone 2 and 5-minute recoveries in zone 1 between sets. These intervals may be done on flat terrain or hills.

Sprint power. This type of advanced-ability training is common in road cycling but unusual in other cycling-related sports. This is because road races often come down to a sprint finish. Workouts at this intensity demand focused motivation in order to fully recruit a large number of muscle units to produce maximal power. In that regard, these sessions are both physically and mentally challenging. An example of a sprint power workout is 5 repeats with each lasting only 10 pedal revolutions at zone 7 with 5-minute recoveries. The terrain can be varied to match what is expected in a given race.

Even though the preceding discussion describes individual workouts for each of these abilities, it is possible and highly recommended that you mix them within a session to more closely simulate the demands of racing. This is very effective during the build period of the season—the last 12 weeks or so before an A-priority race. For example, during a workout you could, after your warm-up, include speed skills drills followed by anaerobic endurance intervals and a steady, long aerobic endurance ride. The possibilities for mixing abilities within a workout are endless, allowing for individual creativity to match your fitness requirements to the demands of an upcoming race.

The only other types of workouts not described in these six categories are those intended to promote recovery and test progress.

Recovery. For the advanced athlete, recovery is generally best accomplished as a low-intensity ride in zone 1. Active recovery has been shown to hasten the return to intense training for veteran riders when compared with passive recovery. It's just the opposite for novices. They are usually better off making the recovery day one completely off the bike. This does not mean that advanced athletes should never take a day off or that novices should never ride easy.

Testing. In order to keep FTP current throughout the training season, you may need to test progress frequently. As mentioned earlier, testing should be done every 4 to 6 weeks following 2 or 3 days of recovery. Of course, as described above, there are other ways to determine FTP without testing. A few back-to-back days of recovery are still beneficial every few weeks even if testing is not performed.

YOU'RE NOW READY to start training with your power meter. All you need to do is set up your power zones using Table 4.1. This assumes you have established your FTP as described earlier in the chapter. If you haven't had an opportunity to do a race or test to determine it, then use the estimation method. This will get you going with the workout types also described in this chapter. If you're anxious to start serious training now, you can skip ahead to the chapter in Part III that applies to your sport. There you will find the details of how to design your training program in order to be fit and fast for your next A-priority race. Should you decide to skip ahead, return to Chapter 5 later; when you do, you will learn how a few more ideas on power can help make your training even more effective so that you race faster.

5

Riding with Intensity

NOW THAT YOU HAVE YOUR TRAINING ZONES set up, you are ready to begin doing workouts based on power. In this chapter, I will take you to the next level of understanding power, which really means understanding intensity.

For the experienced cyclist, intensity must be the focus of training. That doesn't mean that the length of rides is unimportant, only that intensity is more so. If I had to put a number on it, I'd say that intensity accounts for roughly 60 percent of your race fitness, with the remaining 40 percent coming from the length of your rides. How "hard" you train is critical to race performance.

We will examine four ways of better understanding intensity as it relates to power: Intensity Factor, peak power profiles, pacing, and matches. Let's get started by considering how hard your workouts are.

HOW HARD DO YOU RIDE?

For the advanced athlete, the most important element of any training program is intensity. It's not how long the ride is, which is what most athletes rely on as a marker of progress toward greater fitness. How many miles or hours you do in a week has much less impact on your fitness than does the intensity of your individual workouts. Getting the intensity right is much more likely to result in fast racing than simply putting in a lot of "junk" miles.

The reason athletes focus so much on duration as a marker of progress is probably because it's so easily measured; all you need is an odometer or a stopwatch on your bike. Athletes are much less inclined to talk about intensity as a measure of fitness progress as it is far more difficult to measure and define. Here I will show you how you can use power to easily describe intensity so that you can rely on it as a gauge of how your training is going.

Intensity Factor

What if I told you that I did a 90-minute ride at an average power of 200 watts? Would that mean anything to you? Would you know whether that was an easy or a hard ride for me? No, you would not. Without knowing what I am capable of doing, you would not be able to make sense of 200 watts. You would need to compare that number to something else. With a power meter, the standard reference point is Functional Threshold Power. By comparing 200 watts to my FTP, you would know how easy or hard the ride was. And the resulting number would be my Intensity Factor.

Here's how it works. To compare FTP to my 200-watt workout, I could divide the ride's average power by my FTP to find the percentage of FTP at which I rode. For example, let's say my FTP is 350 watts. If I divide 200 by 350, I get 0.571. That means I was riding at 57 percent of my FTP, and 57 percent would be my IF for that session. It was therefore not a particularly hard ride. But if my FTP is 227 watts, the ride was done at 88 percent of FTP (200 ÷ 227 = 0.881). That's a tough workout.

Using IF, you can compare the intensities of workouts or races that you've done, or you can compare them to another rider's. What you will know then is how hard you were riding.

Intensity Factor can also be used in the design of racelike workouts matched to the expected intensity of your A-priority races. Table 5.1 helps you with this by suggesting typical Intensity Factors for common race types. In the 12 weeks before such a race, you should increasingly focus your workouts on the expected race intensity in order to be prepared. Be aware that not all these races are steady-state events in which the IF remains relatively stable throughout. Whereas time trials and triathlons are steady, road and mountain bike races have lots of surges with great changes in intensity throughout. The IF for these races is an average that may include

TABLE 5.1 COMMON RACE INTENSITY FACTORS

RACE TYPE	COMMON INTENSITY FACTOR
IRONMAN (AGE GROUP)	0.60–0.70
IRONMAN (ELITE) HALF-IRONMAN (AGE GROUP)	0.70–0.79
HALF-IRONMAN (ELITE) LONG ROAD RACE MOUNTAIN BIKE MARATHON	0.80–0.89
OLYMPIC AND SPRINT TRIATHLONS LONG TIME TRIAL SHORT MOUNTAIN BIKE RACE	0.90–1.04
SHORT TIME TRIAL	1.05–1.15

extreme highs and lows. This matter of variability will be covered later in this chapter.

Peak Power Profiling

Let's look at another way to describe intensity using power so that it tells you something about how your training and fitness are coming along. In Chapter 3, I told you that power and time are inversely related—when one changes, the other changes in the opposite direction. In other words, an increase in duration causes a decrease in power. You can't stay in zone 7 for more than a few seconds, but you can ride in zone 1 for hours and hours. How long you can stay at a given intensity level says a lot about you as a cyclist.

One rider may be capable of sprinting for a few seconds at a very high intensity—upward of 1,500 watts—while another can manage only half of that sprint power for the same duration. However, the rider with the low-power sprint may be capable of riding for 1 hour at more than 300 watts, while the 1,500-watt sprinter can manage only 250 watts for 1 hour and is dropped long before the finish line.

Power relative to duration is a great marker of fitness and performance. If you can increase your power for a given duration, we can safely say you are more fit for that duration. If your power for a given duration is greater than another rider's for the same duration, then we know who will win a race of that duration (all other things being equal, of course).

The best power you can generate for a given amount of time is called "Peak Power." You have a personal set of Peak Power values for common durations, such as 60 minutes (P60), 30 minutes (P30), 5 minutes (P5), 1 minute (P1), and 6 seconds (P0.1). Likewise, you have a Peak Power for any duration you want to specify. Each of these values is unique to you as an athlete. Just as with FTP, the values change as your fitness changes.

This raises an interesting issue: If each rider has unique Peak Power levels, there must be patterns, or profiles, that define each rider. This profile could tell you the durations at which you are currently best and perhaps even what type of training you need to boost power for a given duration. Perhaps your goal is to race well for 40-km events. That would mean focusing your training on P60 fitness. Or maybe your role on the team is sprinter. Your P0.1 is then critical to your performance. Wouldn't it be nice if you could see this in a chart? What a great tool that would be.

In fact, there is such a chart. It's called a "Power Profile." Each rider has a distinctive profile that helps to define who he or she is as a cyclist. Figures 5.1 and 5.2 show the profiles of two riders with varying Peak Powers. These charts represent their highest power output for every duration over the course of an entire season. To help orient you to these charts, the vertical, or "Y," axis represents power in watts, with zero (0) at the bottom. The horizontal, or "X,"

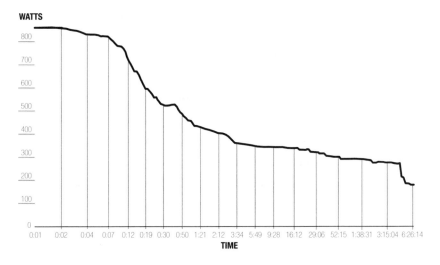

FIGURE 5.1 Power profile for a pro Ironman triathlete

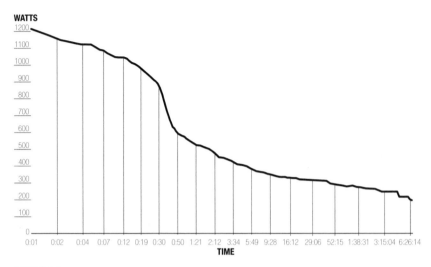

WATTS

FIGURE 5.2 Power profile for a Category III road cyclist

axis, is time, with 1 second on the left end. What you see here for the X axis is a logarithmic, as opposed to a linear, view that places greater emphasis on the shorter durations where most of the changes are likely to occur. Notice that the first 30 minutes comprises about 75 percent of each chart. The higher the line is, the greater the athlete's Peak Power is for that duration.

At first glance, these two charts look quite similar, with power high to the low-duration end on the left and low to the high-duration end on the right. But if you examine the charts in more detail, you'll find some interesting differences that reflect the demands of the sports involved. In Figure 5.1 notice that the male pro triathlete has a 1-second Peak Power of about 860 watts; in Figure 5.2 the male Category III road cyclist shows a 1-second best of about 1,210 watts. The outcomes of Ironman triathlons are never determined by sprint power, but the outcomes of road races often are. The road cyclist trains for this, and it is obvious from his chart.

Notice that on the far right end of the charts, at about 4 hours and 30 minutes, the triathlete's Peak Power is about 270 watts, the roadie's about 250 watts. Again, this reflects the unique demands of the sport. Being capable of riding powerfully for more than 4 hours is what Ironman racing is all about, especially at the pro level.

Another obvious difference on close examination is the shape of the two curves. The roadie's drops off sharply starting at about 30 seconds. For the triathlete the greatest decline occurs at about 7 seconds, but his decline is not nearly as steep.

These differences are probably the result of some natural combination of genetics and training. The exact mix of these ultimate performance determiners is anyone's guess. We can't change genetics, but we can change training. For example, if the pro triathlete in Figure 5.1 decided he wanted to become a road cyclist, he would need to place greater training emphasis on the low-duration end of the chart at the left. That means more short intervals and explosive sprint repeats. He could probably expect that over time his Power Profile would show a change in fitness, with a chart that would begin to look more like the roadie's.

In the same manner, your Power Profile reflects who you are as a cyclist at the current moment, but it is malleable with training. Within the confines of genetics, you can create the fitness you need that is unique to the demands of your races by emphasizing training with appropriate Intensity Factors.

HOW WELL DO YOU PACE?

Pacing is closely related to how you expend your most precious commodity: glycogen. Glycogen is the storage form of carbohydrate, and you have a limited supply. If you're good at replacing expended glycogen stores, you should come to the start line of a race with a full tank. A topped-up glycogen supply will last roughly two hours depending on your unique physiology and how you pace the race. Anything beyond that duration will require the intake of more sugar—sports drinks, bars, gels, blocks, or whatever you like to use. These "exogenous" (outside the body) sources are not as efficiently used by your body as the "endogenous" (inside the body) glycogen stored in your muscles and liver at the start line. When you start running low on your stored endogenous fuel, fatigue begins to set in.

Pacing is also closely related to the body's acidosis. Whenever you increase your power output, your body produces more acid, which limits muscle activity and causes the burning sensation experienced at high intensity. Going above your FTP for an extended time creates a lot of acid, which contributes to the fatigue you experience later in a race—depending, of course, on how well you paced it.

You may have figured out your exact Intensity Factor for the race and therefore what your race power should be. You start the race—a time trial or bike leg of a triathlon—by watching your power and staying in the prescribed range. But then someone catches and passes you, so you speed up briefly. Or you hammer up a hill. This may happen repeatedly throughout the race, with each such episode accompanied by a short surge in power. In addition, you try to maintain goal power on several steep downhills. That's also a surge, as you will see shortly.

Surges waste glycogen and create additional acidosis. By repeatedly speeding up and slowing down, you don't go any faster than if you rode steadily. But those surges needlessly use a lot of glycogen while increasing your blood's acidity. The longer the race is, the greater this two-headed fatigue problem becomes.

You finish the race, however, with about the Intensity Factor range for which you were aiming. So why was the last part of your race slow and painful? Well, despite your average IF being in the proper range (while perhaps on the high end), you didn't pace evenly. You ran low on glycogen and had your muscles swimming in acid in the latter stages of the race. No wonder it was yet another sufferfest.

The problem was not that you raced at the wrong power but that you didn't stay true to that power throughout, owing to constant surges. That brings us to a tool that can help you identify such unsteady riding in what are meant to be steady-state races: the Variability Index™ (VI).

Variability Index

Steady-state races, such as time trials and triathlons, should be ridden . . . well, very steadily. When the race is over, you can determine how steadily you paced the race by checking your VI, which is a comparison of your Normalized Power and average power. Recall that NP is average power normalized to reflect the metabolic cost or sensations of fatigue experienced during a ride. In effect, it gives more value to the power spikes you create. The more spikes in power there are and the bigger the spikes are, the higher the NP is. By comparing NP and average power, you can isolate the spiked portions and therefore know how steadily (or not) you rode. You make this comparison by dividing NP by average power. The result is your VI for a race, a workout, or an interval.

Let's use an example to better understand this. You race in a time trial or triathlon, and afterward, while checking the software or head unit numbers for the race, you see your NP was 256 watts and your average power was 245 watts. That means your VI was 1.04 (256 ÷ 245 = 1.04). Is that good or bad? My general rule of thumb is that for steady-state races your VI should be 1.05 or less. A VI of 1.0 would mean perfect pacing: NP was the same as average power. There were few spikes, and they were small. A VI in excess of 1.05 tells me that you probably wasted a lot of energy by surging and generally not riding steadily.

A while back I received an e-mail from a triathlete who had finished an Ironman the previous weekend. He was disheartened, for even though he had a good bike split time, he had to walk the marathon. "What went wrong?" he asked me. Fortunately, he was using a power meter, so I could look at his race graph. His VI was 1.21. That's what I would expect to see in a 1-hour, hilly criterium. It was much too high for an Ironman bike leg. He was surging frequently throughout the race, wasting energy, and creating lots of acidosis—big-time fatigue! No wonder he walked the marathon.

Variability Index has little relevance to the analysis of nonsteady, variably paced races, such as road races, criteriums, and mountain bike events. By their very nature, they are highly variable. You can't ride steadily without spikes and surges and still be a contender in these races.

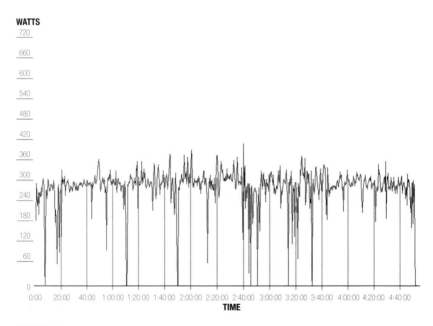

FIGURE 5.3 Example of Variability Index for an Ironman triathlon; VI = 1.04

If you have a low VI, you are just a finisher—or you had a great team protecting you.

Figures 5.3 and 5.4 provide examples of high and low VI from races. In the road race example of Figure 5.4, it's easy to see from all of the power spikes why VI is so high. In contrast, note how small the spikes are and how steadily the Ironman triathlete rode as shown in Figure 5.3.

Steadily Paced Races

When I coach triathletes and time trialists, I devote a great deal of training time to teaching them how to properly pace. Pacing is difficult to master, but it is much easier to do with a power meter than with a heart rate monitor or through the use of perceived exertion. In fact, with power it's almost like cheating. Whereas most athletes in such steady-state events start the race

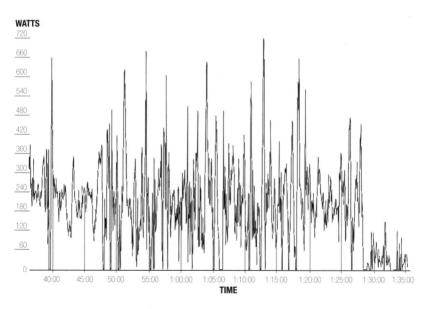

FIGURE 5.4 Example of Variability Index for a road race; VI = 1.31

much too fast, the athlete with a power meter can monitor output, which is much more closely related to performance than is input (see Chapter 1 for a discussion of output and input in racing). All it takes is deciding in advance the power range that you are capable of using during the race to produce the best time. This is determined largely by tracking past experience, by using Intensity Factor, and by knowing your duration-based Peak Power levels from your Power Profile, as described earlier. If it's a 40-km time trial or triathlon and you know it will take you about 1 hour, then you also know that your P60 is about the power you should be aiming for throughout the race. But there's a bit more to it than that since courses typically have small, rolling hills that take a few seconds to go over or even severe climbs lasting several minutes.

A triathlete once asked me what he should do on the downhill portions of an Ironman bike course. Should he pedal hard, pedal easy, or coast? That was a great question and one that gets at the heart of proper pacing on a bike. It has to do with drag—how much wind resistance you encounter as the bike goes faster or slower.

On a bike, as your speed increases linearly (a straight line from, let's say, 20 to 25 mph), the power required to go faster increases exponentially. This is owing primarily to aerodynamic drag from air resistance. So while going from 20 to 25 mph is only a 25 percent increase in speed, there is something like a doubling of the energy required to achieve that additional 5 mph. As speed increases, you must use more energy to sustain that speed, plus additional energy to overcome an increased headwind.

Why am I telling you this? Because as you go downhill and your speed increases, should you want to go even faster than coasting allows, the energy "expense" of the additional miles per hour is going to cost you dearly. If you try to go really fast by pedaling hard downhill, you're going to dip very deeply into your precious carbohydrate stores while causing an increase of hydrogen ions and resulting acidity in your blood. Doing that repeatedly will soon catch up with you. You'll eventually be forced to slow down as a result of wasted energy and acid-bathed muscles. A wasted race.

The bottom line for pacing has to do with an old adage that says that if you are riding on a fast portion of a course (downhill), ride easy, meaning use lower power, but if you are riding on a slow portion of a course (uphill), ride hard, meaning use higher power. So when you ride fast on a downhill, don't expend as much energy as when you ride uphill. Hold back on your power output when going fast. The longer the event is, the more important this is. That is, you can go much harder downhill for a 20-km time trial or a sprint-distance triathlon than for a 40-km time trial or an Ironman.

The best advice I've seen for this concept came from Alan Couzens, an exercise physiologist and triathlon coach. He nailed it with his "50-40-30-20-10 Rule" for Ironman triathletes. The concept applies across all steady-state cycling sports with some possible modification. His rule is described in Table 5.2.

TABLE 5.2   THE 50-40-30-20-10 RULE

IF YOUR GOAL POWER FOR THE RACE IS EXPECTED TO PRODUCE AN AVERAGE SPEED OF ABOUT 30 KPH (19 MPH), THEN . . .	
WHEN YOUR SPEED IS	**YOU SHOULD**
GREATER THAN 50 KPH (31 MPH)	COAST—GET AERO AND STOP PEDALING.
ABOUT 40 KPH (25 MPH)	DECREASE YOUR POWER OUTPUT BELOW GOAL POWER.
ABOUT 30 KPH (19 MPH)	RIDE STEADILY AT GOAL POWER.
ABOUT 20 KPH (12 MPH)	PEDAL A BIT HARDER ABOVE GOAL POWER.
ABOUT 10 KPH (6 MPH)	GO WELL ABOVE GOAL POWER.

SOURCE: Used with permission of Alan Couzens.

Of course, your planned speed may not be 19 mph. The concept, however, remains the same: Conserve energy when the bike is going fast (downhill); expend energy when the bike is going slow (uphill). The numbers in Table 5.2 can be modified to fit your race goals. If your goal is about 25 mph, substitute 40 kph for 30 kph and adjust the others accordingly.

Setting up the table is the easy part. The real key to success is rehearsal. Every time you go for a racelike ride, incorporate the basic concept—ride slightly harder uphill, ride slightly easier downhill, and coast when you are going faster than your upper-end speed on the chart. You'll conserve energy and produce faster bike splits by doing this.

BURNING MATCHES

So far I've explained pacing with power only in steady-state events. Pacing is also critical in variably paced races, such as criteriums and road and mountain bike races—but in an entirely different way.

Matches and Variably Paced Races

In variably paced races, energy expenditure isn't anything like what is common in a time trial or triathlon. Road races, criteriums, and mountain bike races are "variably paced," meaning that your power output will significantly change throughout. Your power at any given moment in such an event depends largely on what others are doing and on the terrain. You can't ride steadily and expect to be a contender in the race. Staying with the group when it speeds up and matching its power surges on climbs are critical to the outcome. As explained above, you should expect to have a high VI in such a race.

That said, it's possible to start too hard in a variably paced race. You are likely to experience a lot of nervous excitement at the start line. When the guns goes off, if you bolt to the front and keep throwing in frequent surges, you'll soon wear yourself out. Controlling your emotions is critical to success in all such races. You don't win a race in the first several minutes, but you can certainly lose it.

Even if you do control your emotions early in the race, some others almost certainly won't. There are going to be many surges as different riders go to the front and drive the pace up. The less experienced the group is with racing, the more likely this is to occur. In the latter portion of the race, there are typically fewer surges, but they are more critical to the outcome.

These surges often last only a few seconds to a couple of minutes at most. They commonly happen when riders are coming out of corners, going up a hill, or attempting to break away from the group. You must be able to respond to these surges, or even initiate them at the right times, if you are to finish well.

Extreme surges are appropriately called "matches" because you get only so many, and once they're gone, they're gone. Given your fitness, you have only a certain number of matches to burn on any given day as you stand at the start line. If you needlessly waste them, you'll have a poor race. But if you burn them in the right amounts at the right moments, you will do well.

The starting place for sound match burnings begins with recognizing that yours are not unlimited and that they can be defined by intensity, duration, and volume: how high the power surge is, how long you maintain it, and how many matches you burn in a race. You can find all of this in postride analysis using WKO+ software. See the sidebar "How to Set Up WKO+ for Matches" for the details.

You can define a match in any way that seems appropriate to you. Here's what I do. For a road race or mountain bike race, I define a match as a surge that lasts 20 seconds or longer with sustained power in zone 7 (see Table 4.1, page 63). For a criterium, I shorten that to 10 seconds in zone 7 as there are likely to be many more short surges that take their cumulative toll on a rider.

The software will find these for you. What you want to know from this search is how many matches you burned, how long they lasted on average, the duration of the longest one, how great their average power was, and what the greatest power was. Armed with this information, you are now able to create workouts that mimic the demands of the race to help you prepare to burn more matches, longer matches, or bigger matches. You will also get a much better sense of how your races are paced, allowing you to be prepared not only physically but also mentally.

HOW TO SET UP WKO+ FOR MATCHES

You can find your matches burned in a race or workout using the WKO+ software feature called "Fast Find." (This feature is found only on WKO+ software.) Here's how to do it.

STEP 1. Open the race graph, and under EDIT in the upper menu select FAST FIND. A pop-up window will appear.

STEP 2. Select the RANGE OF INTEREST you want to check for matches. This could be the entire graph (the whole race) or a selected portion of it.

STEP 3. Set LEADING EDGE by inserting the minimum size of your match in the space labeled "equal to or more than."

STEP 4. For TRAILING EDGE, LESS THAN insert the same number as in step 3.

STEP 5. Set MINIMUM DURATION to the amount of time that defines your match.

STEP 6. Set MAXIMUM DURATION to the longest time you might burn a match. This can be quite long, as in several minutes.

STEP 7. Click on FIND, and bars will appear on your graph for every match that fits your settings. They will also appear as a list of FINDS in the column to the right of the chart. Figure 5.5 shows what this looks like. Here you can also see power, heart rate, and terrain.

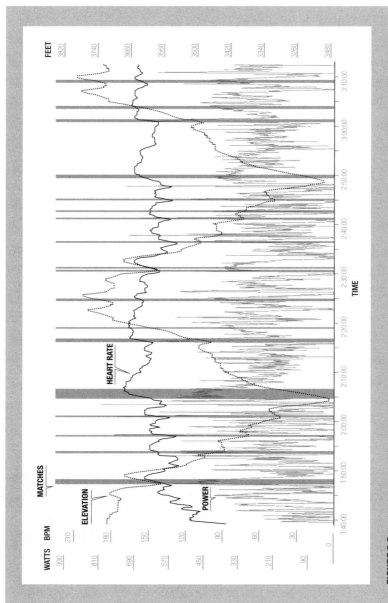

FIGURE 5.5 Matches found in a road race graph (WKO+ software)

Matches and Steady-State Races

It's also possible to burn matches in a time trial or triathlon, but the definition of a match is much more flexible for this type of racing. Although I usually define a match in a variably paced race as being power zone 7, going that intensely in a long, steady race is likely to cause extreme fatigue owing to the glycogen expense and the resulting acidosis. In variably paced races, there are opportunities to recover between surges, but there are no such opportunities in time trials and triathlons. You're riding at your limit for the entire race. Zone 7 surges are likely to result in a "DNF" (did not finish).

In such races, matches are generally needed only on hills and are defined by the duration of the event. The guideline I use is that whenever a time trialist or triathlete exceeds his or her goal power by two or more zones for a certain length of time, a match is being burned. I'll explain. In doing a 40-km race, the rider is likely to be in zone 4 most of the time, so a match would be a brief excursion into zone 6 or higher. A triathlete doing an Ironman in zone 2 would identify a match as zone 4 or higher. The length of the match is a bit harder to define. It's possible to stay in zone 4 for a much longer time than in zone 6.

TABLE 5.3 MATCH SIZE BY ZONE AND DURATION AND CUMULATIVE RACE TIME FOR STEADY-STATE RACES			
RACE GOAL ZONE	ZONE THAT BURNS A MATCH (AND UPPER LIMIT OF INTENSITY)	DURATION IN ZONE THAT BURNS A MATCH (MAY VARY)	RECOMMENDED CUMULATIVE MATCH DURATION FOR RACE (MAY VARY)
ZONE 4	ZONE 6	>1 MINUTE	<5 MINUTES
ZONE 3	ZONE 5	>2 MINUTES	<10 MINUTES
ZONE 2	ZONE 4	>5 MINUTES	<20 MINUTES

Table 5.3 proposes a way of defining the length of a match based on zones and how much time might be accumulated in matches for each given goal zone. Table 4.1 (page 63) can help you decide what "Race Goal Zone" is appropriate for your race type. The column "Recommended Cumulative Match Duration for Race" is only a suggestion. You may well find that you can manage more cumulative match time, or less, when you race in a given power zone. Unfortunately, experience is the only way to determine this. If in doubt, be conservative with how much match time you accumulate in a race.

AS EXPLAINED EARLIER, if you are an experienced rider, intensity is the key to your race performance. Now, armed with such tools as Intensity Factor, peak power profiling, Variability Index, and the concept of matches, you can expand on what you learned in Chapter 4 about training to race. You're now ready for some serious training!

6

Fitter and Faster

ATHLETES TYPICALLY THINK OF TRAINING over the entire course of the season as a way to become more fit for races. I see the season slightly differently. I see training happening in two stages, each with a slightly different purpose.

The first stage is the base period, which encompasses the early part of the season, more than 12 weeks out from the first A-priority race. This is the time to work on general fitness. "General" means training that is not specific to the challenges of the race. You may be doing things, such as lifting weights, that are not exactly what's demanded of you in the race.

The second stage is the build period. It makes up most of the last 12 weeks prior to the race. This is when general fitness is converted to race-specific readiness. You are now training to become faster, not just fitter.

This distinction may seem trivial, but it really isn't. There are lots of things going on in the build period that have little or no impact on physiological measures of fitness, such as pacing control, equipment selection, and terrain familiarization. What was only general fitness in the base period becomes race-specific preparation to go fast in the build period. In this chapter, we'll examine base period fitness and build period "fastness," and we'll see how your power meter can help you get the most from both periods.

BASE PERIOD: DEVELOPING FITNESS

In Chapter 4, I told you about the six abilities that define training: aerobic endurance, muscular force, speed skills, muscular endurance, anaerobic endurance, and sprint power. The first three are the most basic and determine the level of your fitness for the remainder of the year. They must be well developed by the end of the base period.

By far the most important of the six abilities for the endurance athlete is aerobic endurance. Before you start training to become faster and race ready in the build period, you must be aerobically fit, and building aerobic fitness is the primary purpose of the base period. So how do you know when aerobic endurance, and therefore your readiness to train to race fast, is at a high point? Your power meter and software can help answer this question. They will help you keep track of two important markers. I call the first one the "Efficiency Factor (EF)" and the second one "decoupling."

Efficiency Factor

In Chapter 3, I described the relationship between heart rate and power. You may recall that as your aerobic fitness improves, your power increases while your heart rate remains constant. This means that at the start of the season, you may be riding along in heart rate zone 2 and at the same time be in power zone 2. But later in the season, when your fitness is greater, you may still be in heart rate zone 2 while riding in power zone 3. This shifting of power relative to heart rate presents a unique opportunity to measure change in aerobic fitness.

If your power increases at any aerobic intensity (below your lactate threshold), that is certainly a good thing. It means you can now go faster than before even though effort stays the same. This takes us back to the output-input discussion in Chapter 1. *Output* is your productivity—what you are accomplishing. This is your power in watts. *Input* is your effort—how hard you are working. That's your heart rate in beats per minute. Comparing output and input—in other words, comparing power and heart rate—tells you how efficiently you are riding. It's the same as talking about the efficiency rating of your car: how many miles (output) it gets per gallon of gas (input).

Now let's apply this concept to measure your aerobic endurance fitness progress, especially in the base period when this is a critical training ability. Once aerobic fitness is well developed, you can move on to the next period of training, when your workouts become more racelike. Prior to power meters, there was no way of knowing when it was time to make this transition. The rider or coach had to make assumptions about how the rider's aerobic endurance was coming along based only on perceived changes and past experience. But now you can measure this quite precisely. I'll show you how using Efficiency Factor.

Aerobic endurance workouts. EF establishes the ratio of power to heart rate for a given type of ride. This can be done for any aerobic workout. Early in the season, I like to use heart rate zone 2 as this is usually the zone in which most riders are at their aerobic (not *an*aerobic) threshold. All you do is warm up briefly and then ride steadily for a set amount of time in heart rate zone 2. You can ride anywhere from as little as 30 minutes to as much as 4 hours. (Longer races require longer rides, so you would set your ride time in accordance with your targeted A-priority race.) Pay no attention to your power.

When you've finished the ride, divide your Normalized Power by average heart rate for the zone 2 portion of the ride. The result is your EF. (If you use TrainingPeaks.com for analysis, this calculation will be made automatically; EF may be found on the workout graph display.)

By comparing the resulting ratios for similar workouts over several weeks, you can measure improvements in aerobic efficiency. To be reliable, your workouts need to be quite similar, which means that you need to make sure all of the variables are similar. The list of variables includes level of pre-workout fatigue, equipment, course, weather conditions, altitude, pre-workout nutrition (especially stimulants such as caffeine, which affects heart rate), warm-up, and perhaps even time of day. The more similar all of these are from one session to the next, the more valuable the information is.

You can also do this workout by keeping power constant and then seeing what happens to your heart rate when finished. If you choose this method, be sure to do it that way every time. I do it the other way around because there is research showing that heart rate may decrease when the rider is fatigued. Seeing the decrease in heart rate would certainly give a false impression of improvement. But there is no research I've ever seen showing that power increases with fatigue, which is why I believe making heart rate the constant is a bit safer.

Also, should you decide to make power the constant, don't use zones. Instead, use a standard wattage that corresponds with your zone 2 power at the start of the base period. If you decide to use zone 2 power as your constant and your FTP changes in the base period (as it should), then your zones will also change. So you may be riding at a higher power output, which would make comparisons with previous EF data useless.

TABLE 6.1 EXAMPLES OF WEEKLY EFFICIENCY FACTORS FROM ZONE 2 AEROBIC THRESHOLD WORKOUTS IN THE EARLY BASE PERIOD

DATE	EFFICIENCY FACTOR
DEC. 23	1.63
DEC. 30	1.67
JAN. 6	1.70
JAN. 13	1.87
JAN. 20	1.76
JAN. 27	1.88
FEB. 3	1.90
FEB. 10	1.87

If you are making good aerobic progress, your EF will rise over the course of a few weeks in the base period. Table 6.1 shows examples for an athlete I coached of his EF from weekly rides done in the lower half of heart rate zone 2 for an 8-week base period. Each of the rides was done for 2 hours.

Note how steadily his EF rose in the first four weeks. This shows a good response to training. His aerobic endurance fitness was definitely improving. In the fifth week, there was a setback as EF dropped to 1.76 from the previous week's high of 1.87. This is not unusual. In fact, such setbacks often happen frequently. Don't be concerned about one or two negative test results. If the numbers drop repeatedly, however, you may want to check to make sure the variables listed above are in order.

Looking at Table 6.1 further, you can see that in the last three weeks the changes in EF became smaller and essentially leveled off. This leveling is a good sign that aerobic endurance fitness is at a peak level and that this rider is ready to move on to more challenging workouts, including tempo rides.

Sweet-spot workouts. Dr. Andrew Coggan, who developed many power-training concepts, calls workouts performed at 88 to 93 percent of FTP the "sweet spot" because this particular range is especially good for building FTP. I use the same method for sweet-spot rides as I do for aerobic workouts, only now the workout is performed as long intervals instead of as a steady state. I have the rider warm up and then do 20-minute intervals in high power zone 3 and low power zone 4 with 5-minute recoveries in power zone 1.

This sweet-spot workout is classified as muscular endurance owing to the zone 4 intensity, but it is really an advanced aerobic endurance workout. I typically use it once I see the EF from zone 2 beginning to stabilize (as seen in the last three weeks in the Table 6.1 example). There may be an overlap of a few weeks between aerobic endurance and sweet-spot workouts. Again, be sure to control the variables that may affect the outcome.

Contrary to what we've been led to believe in old training lore, zone 3 is very effective for improving aerobic fitness and FTP. I have a rider do only 2 of these 20-minute intervals in a workout. Later on, in the last 12 weeks before the race, such as a half-Ironman or Ironman triathlon, I'll have the athlete do 3 to 6 zone 3 intervals in a single session in the same manner since these are close to being racelike for such events.

Determining EF from an interval session takes a bit of time and a calculator. Add the Normalized Power for the intervals and divide by the number of intervals to find the average interval NP. Do the same for heart rate for each interval. Now divide the average interval NP by the average interval heart rate to find EF for the sweet-spot portion of the session.

Table 6.2 provides examples of EF from sweet-spot workouts. Note once more that there may occasionally be negative progress, as seen here in the week of February 6. This is to be expected. Press on with your training, but

TABLE 6.2 EXAMPLES OF WEEKLY EFFICIENCY FACTORS FROM SWEET-SPOT WORKOUTS IN THE LATE BASE PERIOD

DATE	EFFICIENCY FACTOR
JAN. 23	1.60
JAN. 30	1.70
FEB. 6	1.64
FEB. 13	1.75
FEB. 20	1.77

be doubly careful about controlling as many variables as possible. When EF begins to stabilize for this workout, you know that your aerobic fitness has reached another high, probably along with an increased FTP, and you are ready to go on to even more advanced training.

Decoupling

Decoupling is a second way to gauge aerobic endurance and is accomplished by measuring the output-input relationship changes that take place during a workout or race. It provides guidance on how aerobically fit you are from a single ride instead of collecting data over several sessions. For this metric to provide useful information, the workout or segment must have been fully aerobic (below the lactate threshold) and steady (Variability Index of 1.05 or less). It's a somewhat less reliable marker than EF as so many things can affect heart rate during rides of varying types. But I've found it good for giving snapshots of whether your aerobic endurance fitness is really sound. It takes a fair amount of calculating, but if you are using TrainingPeaks.com or WKO+ software, the hard work is done for you. Both indicate decoupling as the metric "Pw:HR" found on the workout graph page.

The software compares Efficiency Factors for the two halves of the workout or selected workout segment (such as an interval or a steady-state portion). The difference between EF for the first half and EF for the second is divided by EF for the first half. This produces a percentage of increase or decrease in EF for the second half. Basically, what this number is telling you is how much your heart rate or power drifted during the ride. Large amounts of drift are common when fitness is poor.

Any change in the relationship between power and heart rate is decoupling. In the accompanying Figures 6.1 through 6.4, you can see how heart rate and power are sometimes parallel or nearly so (coupled) or obviously not parallel at all (decoupled).

For aerobic workouts that are fairly steady but not necessarily tightly controlled (as in aerobic endurance rides), I like to see athletes achieve a

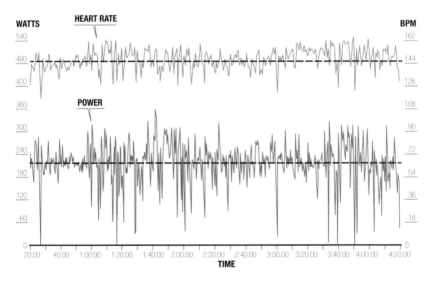

FIGURE 6.1 A 4-hour ride in heart rate zone 2 following a 20-minute warm-up, with 3 percent decoupling (aerobic endurance quite good)

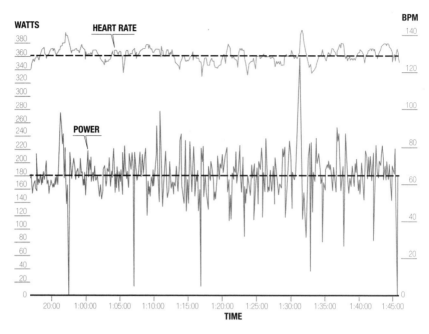

FIGURE 6.2 A 2-hour aerobic endurance ride, with 2 percent decoupling (sound aerobic endurance)

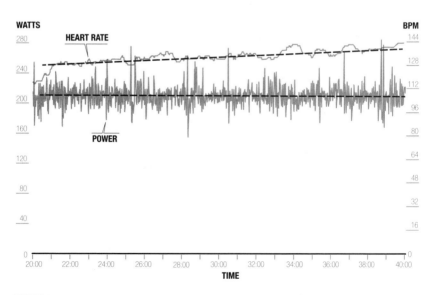

FIGURE 6.3 A 20-minute ride in power zone 3 following a 20-minute warm-up, with 5 percent decoupling in a short duration (questionable aerobic endurance)

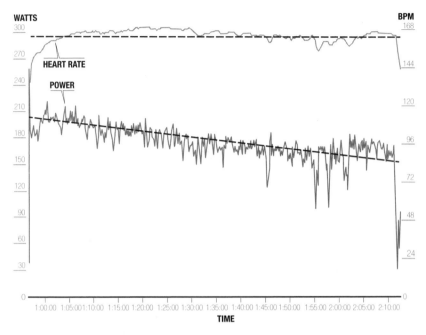

FIGURE 6.4 A steady 2-hour ride in heart rate zone 3 following a 1-hour warm-up, with 8 percent decoupling (poor aerobic endurance)

decoupling of 5 percent or less. You may occasionally see negative numbers. These are, of course, less than a positive 5 percent and may reflect outside variables such as warm-up and weather but may be assumed to be good results. As with EF, there are many variables that affect heart rate and therefore decoupling, such as heat, caffeine, and rested state. These variables must be controlled whenever possible for decoupling to be indicative of aerobic status.

Generally speaking, an athlete's aerobic endurance is sound if decoupling is consistently 5 percent or less for steady-state aerobic workouts. For example, if you quit training for a while, your decoupling will reflect your loss of fitness. This will be obvious as an increase in fatigue late in the workout; the fatigue will either cause your heart rate to rise or your power to drop off—or both. In either case, decoupling of greater than 5 percent indicates an acutely low level of aerobic endurance fitness.

BUILD PERIOD: PREPARING TO RACE FAST

Following the base period of your season, general fitness should be quite well established. By this point in the season, your FTP should be higher than it was a few weeks before and your aerobic endurance, as indicated by Efficiency Factor and decoupling, should be high and relatively stable. This should all be in place 12 weeks prior to your A-priority race. If it is, then you are fit. Now it's time to become race ready and faster. To do that, your training must increasingly match the demands of your projected race.

As I'm sure you are aware by now, there are only two elements of race readiness to worry about: duration and intensity. In the old days, race training was all about miles and effort. Now that you have a power meter, however, it's primarily TSS and IF.

In this last 12 weeks before the A-priority race, the basic factors that describe how specific individual training sessions relate to the demands of racing are workout Intensity Factor, Training Stress Score, match burning, and proper pacing. As this specific-preparation portion of the season progresses, your workouts should increasingly meet the TSS, IF, match-burning, and pacing demands of your A-priority race. If they do, then you are becoming race ready. This is the most basic way of determining if you are doing the right types of workouts.

The most important portions of the race are determined and rehearsed in training. In triathlon these are usually hilly sections. Hills are also critical determiners of race outcomes in a road or mountain bike race, but success in these events also has a lot to do with the actions of other riders. This implies the need for group rides that simulate critical portions of the race. Let's take a look at how two athletes I coached, a road racer and a triathlete, prepared for the specific demands of their races.

Road Race-Specific Workout

Figure 6.5 is a graph of a workout done on the USAC Masters Nationals Road Race course by one of the athletes I coached. Here you see only the hard portion of the ride following the warm-up. He did this workout 6 days prior to the race during his peak period, so the hard portion was restricted to about 1 hour. This workout would have been a more racelike experience had it been done with a group of riders, but such a group was not available at the time. However, before he arrived for the race, he had ridden with groups on hilly courses similar to what he expected on race day.

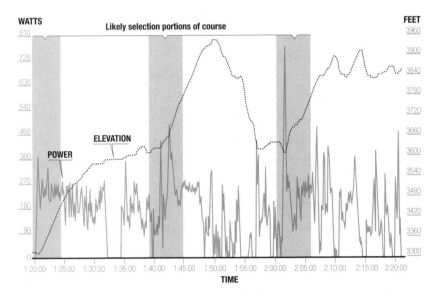

FIGURE 6.5 Preparing for the demands of a road race by training on a portion of the course with racelike intensities at the anticipated selection points (the section shown in this workout graph was done twice in the race)

Figure 6.5 shows the elevation change and power output during the racelike workout. The section of the course you see here was covered twice in the race. We had identified three likely selection points on each lap (places where the race was likely to break apart), based primarily on terrain but also on position in the race relative to the finish line. The purpose of the ride was to rehearse the anticipated race intensities at these points.

It turned out that we were right about when attempts to break up the peloton would be attempted. The rider said it was his best road race ever. Our success was owing to diligent preparation.

Triathlon-Specific Workout

Figure 6.6 is a triathlete's graph for an Olympic-distance (40-km) race. The graph shows power and elevation. Hills played a significant role in this race even though they were not terribly steep or long. The two most critical areas, which are highlighted, were 800 to 1,200 meters long, with grades of about 4 percent.

The rider did not have access to the course for training prior to race day, so she found similar hills near her home. A portion of the race preparation involved doing weekly repeats on these hills at planned race power. That race power level was greater than the planned, overall Normalized Power for the entire race and was based on the 50-40-30-20-10 Rule (see Table 5.2, page 83), along with controlling for matches burned (see Table 5.3, page 88). I knew that she could manage the flat sections of the course, but athletes commonly work too hard on hills. The frequent hill repeats workouts got her ready for that.

The planned Intensity Factor of 90–95 percent for the race would put her in zone 4 for most of it. So in the last 12 weeks prior to race day, she did weekly muscular endurance intervals in zone 4. Racing in this zone means climbing in zones 5 and 6 for a triathlon or time trial. She trained to stay in these zones for the duration of each climb knowing that the upper

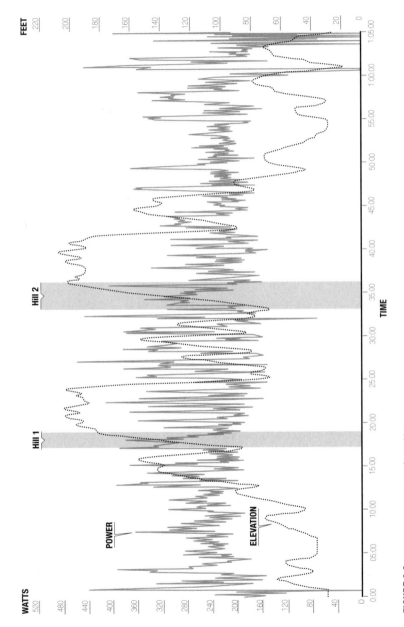

FIGURE 6.6 Preparing for the demands of a triathlon

limit (zone 6) should not be maintained for longer than about 1 minute. We anticipated that the first climb would take about 2 minutes and the second about 4 minutes. We found similar hills near her house and used them for rehearsal in training.

On race day, there was nothing new other than the butterflies in her stomach. Without a power meter, she would have been at the mercy of her emotions throughout the race, especially in the first several minutes and on each of the climbs. With a plan built around power, however, managing intensity was easy. She gauged intensity precisely throughout the ride. Her Variability Index for the bike portion of the race was 1.05, also indicative of a race that was well paced.

ARE YOU FITTER AND FASTER?

As I've mentioned a few times now, over the course of the season your training should progress from an emphasis on general-fitness preparation to a focus on race-specific preparation. The general-fitness training of the base period is primarily directed at improving aerobic endurance. Once that is well developed, you are ready to advance beyond base by training to race faster. Doing so may include training strategies to enhance pace management, climbing, sprint power, and anaerobic capacity to produce bigger and longer-lasting matches. Other, non-power-related concerns as you shift toward race-specific training include knowledge of your competitors and their typical race styles, race plan creation, race-day nutrition refinement, mental preparedness, and equipment selection.

Effective training means watching for markers of change in many areas. The following are some of the power markers from workout analysis over the course of a season that serve as indicators that your training is paying off as you move from becoming fitter to becoming faster.

FTP Changes

The most basic way to gauge progress toward greater fitness and faster racing is to monitor changes in your FTP. Hopefully the changes are positive. FTP should be rising throughout the base period. It may even continue to rise in the last 12 weeks before your A-priority race. But you may not see much change in the build period if you saw rapid and significant upward shifts in FTP during the base period. That's okay; the emphasis is now on becoming faster, which doesn't always involve changes in FTP. There are many other power indicators of change that point toward greater race readiness.

Power Distribution Changes

An indirect indicator that training is progressing from general fitness in the base period to race specificity in the build period is the shift in training time spent in each power zone. Figure 6.7 shows the power distribution by zones for a cyclist who does mostly road races. Figure 6.8 illustrates the same for a triathlete who focuses on the half-Ironman distance. Notice that in the base period, there is very little difference between the power distributions by zones for the two sports. In fact, this similarity is common across all endurance sports. The base period, especially the early base period, is almost always focused heavily on zone 2 training.

And that holds true here. Both the roadie and the triathlete are concentrating their training on aerobic endurance training with lots of zone 2. But by the build period, the differences are impressive. The road cyclist is spending a great deal more time training in the upper zones (4 through 7), whereas the triathlete is concentrating on zones 2 and 3. Both are doing what is right for their sports in the last 12 weeks of training by making their workouts increasingly racelike. This is reflected by their power distribution. As mentioned before, the outcomes of road races are often determined by

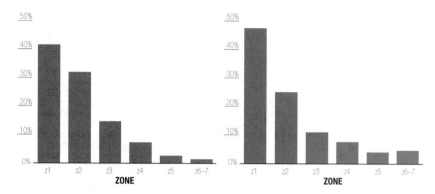

FIGURE 6.7 Power distribution by zones (z) for a road cyclist in the base (left) and build (right) periods

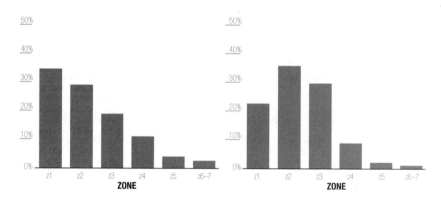

FIGURE 6.8 Power distribution by zones (z) for a triathlete in the base (left) and build (right) periods

what happens in very brief episodes lasting a few seconds to a couple of minutes. This requires high power output. Half-Ironman triathlons, by contrast, are raced by most age-group athletes in power zone 3.

So the demands of your targeted race determine how you train in the last 12 weeks. The most basic question to answer is "In what zones will you be racing?" Knowing the answer to that question then defines the focus of your training in the build period. Table 4.1 (page 63) can help you determine this information.

Watts per Kilograms Changes

We can talk about your power as either absolute or relative. *Absolute* means the highest numbers you can produce regardless of any other factors. Your FTP is an example of this. *Relative* means as compared with something, such as your body weight. I'll explain absolute power as a race-readiness marker in the next section. But for now let's look at power relative to your body weight.

How much you weigh is significant when it comes to going up hills. It takes more absolute power for a heavy rider to climb a hill at a given speed than for a light rider. I expect that is obvious. As a thought experiment, imagine putting on a 50-pound backpack and then riding up a familiar hill. There should be no doubt that it would require a much greater effort on your part to make it to the top in whatever your normal time is for that hill. Take off the backpack, try the climb again, and notice how you seem to be flying uphill. Conversely, going down a hill with the backpack on would make you faster. Now gravity is your friend.

Weight is indeed important when gravity plays a major role in performance. But when gravity is less important to outcome, as when you are riding on flat terrain, being heavier can be an advantage. Let's take a look at why this is so.

A major determiner of climbing performance is watts per kilogram. At these times, how much power you can generate relative to body weight often decides timed results. On flat terrain, however, performance is largely determined by power per unit of aerodynamic drag. And since there is little difference in the drag of a small rider and a large one when they are both in an aero position, the large rider has an advantage. That's because, if nothing else, a large rider typically has a heavier leg with more muscle than a smaller rider. That usually means a higher FTP. So the large rider, who can produce more absolute power, has a definite advantage when the terrain is flat. But when it's uphill, power relative to body weight is crucial to the outcome.

A 176-pound rider may create 5 percent more drag than a 132-pound rider, but the heavier rider is much stronger and can therefore drive a higher gear. On a flat course, absolute power is king. In terms of gravity, however, the large rider weighs 33 percent more and so has a definite disadvantage on a hill. Going uphill demands high power relative to weight. If all other factors were the same (for example, fitness and equipment) and these two riders raced uphill, I'd put my money on the smaller one.

How much power you can generate on a hill is expressed in terms of watts per kilogram of body weight (w/kg). This is a better indicator of climbing ability than absolute power because it includes the crucial measurement of body weight.

To determine your watts per kilogram, first divide your weight in pounds by 2.2. For example, the 176-pound rider's weight in kilograms is 80, and the 132-pounder's is 60. Next, plug in your FTP. Using our example, let's assume the larger rider's FTP is 330 watts. That means when climbing his w/kg is 4.1 ($330 \div 80 = 4.1$). If the smaller rider's FTP is 265, then she is climbing at 4.4 w/kg and so will climb faster—again, if we assume that all other factors are equal and that both riders are climbing at their FTP. So even though her absolute power is about 20 percent less, she climbs faster because her power relative to body weight is about 7 percent greater.

The bottom line here is that to improve as a climber, you need to increase power or decrease weight. The excess weight doesn't need to be body weight; it can be equipment weight. One extra pound of baggage, regardless of its source, takes roughly 1.5 additional watts to get it up a hill. Since endurance athletes commonly have lost a little bit of weight by the time they enter the build period, climbing improvement can be expected. The same thing would happen if weight stayed the same and absolute power increased. That's where we go next.

Peak Power Changes

In Chapter 5, I introduced the concept of Peak Power. Recall that this has to do with your best wattage for given periods of time, such as 30 minutes (P30), 1 minute (P1), or any other measure of time. In that chapter, we used Peak Power from 1 second to several hours to create a Power Profile chart showing how a rider's best absolute power values can be used to graphically illustrate what type of rider he or she is. Also in Chapter 5, I showed you the Power Profiles of a pro triathlete and a Category III road cyclist. In the following section, I'll describe how to gauge your Power Profile changes as you become race ready. But for now let's take a look at how Peak Power can be used as a marker of race readiness.

One of the best indicators of your preparedness to perform well in a certain type of race is how much absolute power you can generate for periods of time that are predictive of the demands of your race. For example, road races are often determined by very brief episodes lasting only a few seconds to a few minutes. If your P1 is increasing as you approach race day, that's a great indicator of your readiness for that type of race. In the same way, if a triathlete's or mountain biker's P30 is increasing, he or she can feel assured that training is going as it should.

Keeping track of changes in your Peak Power is a great way, perhaps the ultimate way, to measure race readiness. There's no doubt that becoming more powerful, especially in the ranges that are critical to success in your event, is an excellent marker of your preparedness.

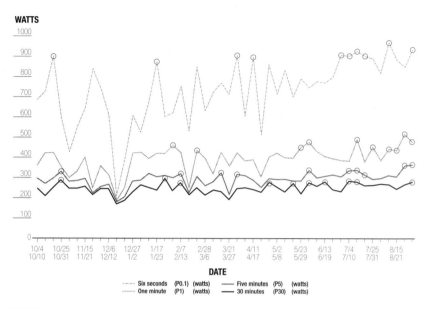

WATTS

DATE

Six seconds (P0.1) (watts) — Five minutes (P5) (watts)
One minute (P1) (watts) — 30 minutes (P30) (watts)

FIGURE 6.9 Peak power by week showing top 10 values in each category (circled) for a masters road cyclist

Figures 6.9 and 6.10 show the top 10 Peak Power values for a road cyclist and a triathlete. Both race at the masters level. The road cyclist's Peak Powers are shown for 6 seconds, 1 minute, 5 minutes, and 30 minutes. All are important durations for successful road racing. The triathlete's Peak Powers are the same except for the absence of 6 seconds, which is inconsequential to the outcome of a triathlon. We could actually make a similar argument for omitting 1 minute for the triathlete, but I left it in just for comparison's sake. Let's start with the roadie in Figure 6.9.

The circles in these figures represent the rider's best 10 power outputs at each duration for the season up to that point. So having the circles move to the right is a very good thing because it means that power is improving. Clusters of circles are great indications that the athlete is coming to a high

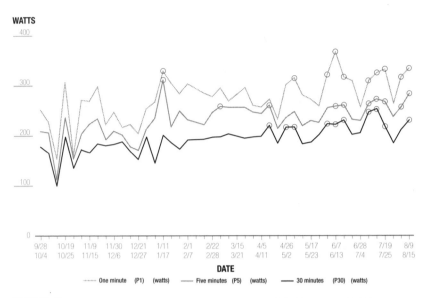

WATTS

.... One minute (P1) (watts)   —— Five minutes (P5) (watts)   —— 30 minutes (P30) (watts)

DATE

FIGURE 6.10 Peak power by week showing top 10 values in each category (circled) for a masters triathlete

point for race readiness. These clusters usually will begin to appear shortly before important races. Half of the circles on this chart appear in the most recent 9 weeks. So this athlete is currently quite well prepared to race. That was obviously not the case on the left side of the chart, early in the season. There are very few circles and no clusters.

The triathlete's current race status is even better, as shown in Figure 6.10. In the last 11 weeks, nearly all the top 10 Peak Powers occurred at each duration. It's just one big cluster to the right side. Now is the time to race.

Power Profile Changes

With WKO+ software or TrainingPeaks.com, you can set up your Power Profile, as described in Chapter 5, to compare the Peak Powers of the current season with those from the previous one or from any other segments of time, such as the present season's base and build periods. I find this a particularly helpful way of seeing how much progress is made over time. Seeing the power changes taking place relative to how you were doing previously is great feedback on progress toward your race goals.

These changes represent improvements in endurance or, said another way, decreases in fatigue. As any section of the Power Profile that is important to you improves (meaning that it rises relative to a previous profile), your endurance and resistance to fatigue are improving. Figures 6.11 through 6.14 show the changes occurring in the Power Profiles of a road cyclist from the previous season (solid lines) to the present one (dashed lines). These are, essentially, four snapshots of the progress he has been making in the current season. Figure 6.11 is his Profile as it looked in January. Figure 6.12 is his Profile in April of the same year. A month later, in May, his Profile changes are shown in Figure 6.13. And, finally, near the end of his race season in August, we see his Profile in Figure 6.14.

By comparing any given duration across the horizontal, or X, axis, we can see how his race readiness is improving. For examples of this, let's examine the changes taking place in both the very brief durations of a few seconds on the left end and the longer durations of several hours on the right end.

This cyclist did a lot of criteriums, and so his sprint power was important. That can be seen in the changes that take place on the left side of the chart. A good example of this is Figure 6.13, where the rider's power for 4 seconds has risen well above where it was for the previous season. It isn't until May (Figure 6.13) that there are significant changes in his sprint power. In May, although he isn't producing any more power for 1 second (about 1,080 watts) than previously, his 4-second power has increased from about 900 watts to about 1,020. That means he could then hold a high-power sprint

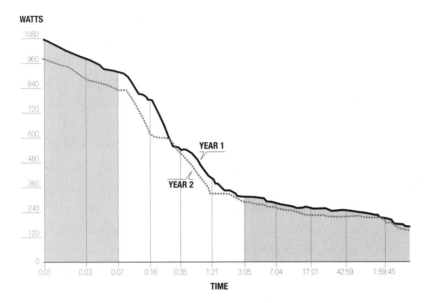

FIGURE 6.11 Power profile in January

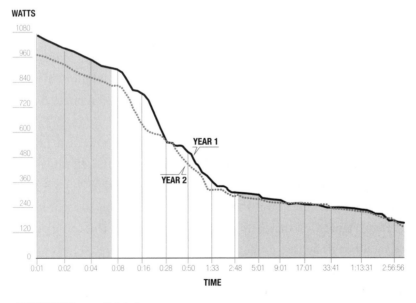

FIGURE 6.12 Power profile in April

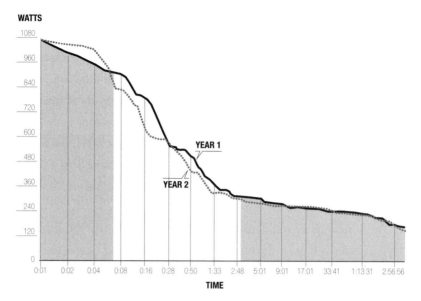

FIGURE 6.13 Power profile in May

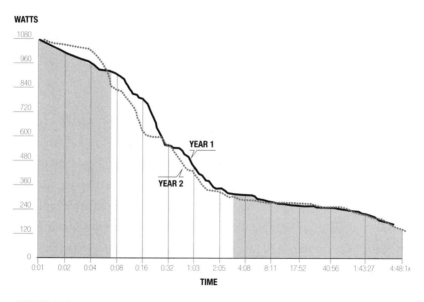

FIGURE 6.14 Power profile in August

for a longer period of time than previously. This change results from training in ways that stressed his power production at the longer duration. It has obvious implications for his racing when a long sprint may determine the outcome. This did not change in the last 3 months of the season.

Notice that by April his power on the right end of the chart has risen to the same level it was when at the highest the previous season. This reflects an emphasis on long-duration training during the base period. From April until August, there are no further changes.

In the same way, we could take any other critical section of the chart for the type of races you do and compare progress. This could be a season-to-season comparison as shown in these figures. Or you may prefer to see the changes taking place between two periods of the current season by comparing, for example, the base and build periods. You could also examine the final 12-week buildup to an important race with your progression before a previous race. The options are nearly endless and provide a great tool for gauging how you are progressing relative to another known period of time.

YOU SHOULD NOW HAVE a solid understanding of what you need to accomplish in the base and build periods. Your power meter and its software will help you refine your training and gauge the progress of both general fitness and race-specific fastness. You certainly made the right decision in purchasing a power meter. I know it was expensive, but it's a remarkable tool that will help take your race preparation to a higher level in ways nothing else can. In the next chapter, we'll take a look at how you can improve your performance even more by mastering a few new ways of thinking about training from a power perspective.

7

Using Your Power Meter for High Performance

THIS CHAPTER IS FOR THE ADVANCED ATHLETE or coach who is focused on two or three A-priority races in a season with the intent of producing a peak performance in each. Here we will be looking at a way to manage preparation for high performance that is on the cutting edge of training science. It's deep stuff.

If you are new to training and racing, this chapter may be well beyond your need for understanding how to use your power meter. The deep stuff, however, doesn't begin to show up until we get to the section titled "Power and Periodization." If peak performance is not your thing—if you're riding and racing strictly for fun—then I'd still strongly recommend reading everything up to that point. You'll come away with a better understanding of training. Of course, you can start into the more advanced parts that come later in the chapter and stop at any time. Then perhaps at some time in the future, when you are giving serious thought to a peak performance and have your power meter and its software pretty well figured out, you can return to this chapter and read it all.

Here we go into the future of training for truly serious athletes.

POWER-TRAINING COMPONENTS

There are three components that taken together define what training is all about. They are frequency, duration, and intensity. It doesn't matter if you are a pro who races in the Tour de France or a green novice just trying to get into decent riding shape; these are the only aspects of your workout routine that can be changed. I'm sure this is not news to you. It's training 101. What I'm going to do here is build on this basic starting point so that by the end of this chapter you will be able to use these concepts along with your power meter and software to produce peak performance for an important race on a specific day. But first let's make sure that we are in agreement on the three components of training.

Frequency

Frequency is nothing more than how often you ride. This is the most basic component of training.

For the novice cyclist, how often he or she rides is the greatest determinant of fitness. Just getting on the bike frequently and riding, regardless of how long or how hard, are the key. This, of course, doesn't mean riding at high intensities or for long durations. With frequent rides at comfortable intensities and manageable durations, the novice will see steady improvement.

Frequency is also important for experienced athletes, just not as important as for the novice. You can't regularly miss workouts, however, and expect to become fitter and faster at any level as an athlete. If you become lackadaisical about working out and the number of rides you do in a week decreases, significant amounts of fitness are eventually lost. At the highest levels, road cyclists and mountain bikers typically ride at least 6 days a week. That saddle-time consistency has a lot to do with their performance. Interestingly, going from 6 to 7 workouts in a week won't have much of an impact on fitness. But decreasing frequency from 6 to 5 will cause a noticeable loss of fitness for the advanced rider. I know that doesn't sound fair. It's just the way fitness seems to work, I've found.

Training frequency is a great challenge for triathletes. Experienced triathletes typically ride a bit less than experienced roadies or mountain bikers. They are generally on their bikes only 4 or 5 times a week in order to make time for swim and run sessions. The optimal use of limited training time is the greatest conundrum facing multisporters, especially in bike training since the bike leg accounts for about half of one's finish time over a standard triathlon race distance. For example, if a triathlete finishes an Olympic-distance race in 2 hours, the bike split is roughly 1 hour. For a 12-hour Ironman triathlon, the bike leg is usually completed in around 6 hours. With this in mind, I highly recommend that triathletes spend roughly half of their weekly training time on the bike.

Frequency is a critical component of effective training whether you use a power meter or not. It accounts for half of what we call "volume"—the total number of hours or miles you train in a week. The other half of volume comes from workout duration.

Duration

How long should you ride? The answer varies according to the kind of events you do. Advanced athletes doing long road races, Ironman triathlons, mountain bike marathons, and centuries typically do one or more of their weekly rides in excess of 4 hours. This helps to prepare them for the rigors of a long race. If the targeted event is shorter, it's typical for the length of the longest rides to also decrease. Of course, regardless of race distance, there are likely to be shorter active recovery rides (done in zone 1), which help the athlete bounce back from the previous day's long or hard ride. Between the longest ride and the recovery rides are workouts that focus generally on higher intensity.

Intensity

For the experienced cyclist, training is mostly about intensity. Sport science research has repeatedly shown this to be true. If all you do as an experienced athlete is ride long sessions at low intensity with an emphasis on weekly volume, you will never achieve anything near your potential in sport. How important is intensity? If I had to put a number on it, I'd say that intensity accounts for about 60 percent of your fitness. Most of the remaining portion comes from the duration of your key workouts. Weekly volume is a distant third.

This doesn't necessarily mean training at the highest intensity possible but rather training with an emphasis on riding at about race intensity, especially in key workouts. A key workout is one intended to challenge and therefore improve some aspect of your fitness related to the six training abilities described in Chapter 4. The hardest key workout is always one that closely simulates both the duration and the intensity of the event. It's also the workout most likely to prepare you for the rigors of your race. Do not sacrifice intensity of such a workout simply to ride longer. It's not a good trade-off.

Workload

Workload is the sum of frequency, duration, and intensity. It can be expressed for a single workout as the combination of duration and intensity or, for a given period of time, such as a week, as a blend of all of three.

For a single workout, as either duration or intensity increases or decreases, your session workload also increases or decreases. Long rides at a low intensity can produce the same workload as short rides at high intensity. This doesn't mean that the resulting fitness is the same. Fitness is a separate matter having to do with how specifically the duration and intensity of workouts are designed relative to the targeted race. But the session workload can be the same no matter what mix of duration and intensity is used.

Weekly workload is the combined result of a week's volume (frequency + duration) and intensity. Athletes tend to think of workload strictly in terms of volume: how many hours or miles in a week. Based on what I've told you, that is hardly the best way to describe workload because it leaves out the most important ingredient: intensity. It's not how many miles but what you do with those miles that makes the most difference on race day.

Workload can be determined for a day, a week, a month, a year, or any other unit of time, such as a training block. Knowing your total workload for a given time allows you to better manage your training and therefore your race performance. By increasing the workload, you can improve fitness; by decreasing it, you can recover. So how do you combine volume and intensity to put a number on your workload? That's where a power meter once again can provide a solution.

Training Stress Score

Hard training causes stress. In fact, stress is what good training is all about. When your body experiences training stress, it responds by first becoming fatigued. Then, usually within hours and given adequate recovery, it begins to adapt to the new level of stress. We call this adaptation "fitness." After a single stressful workout, this new level of fitness is so minute it can't be measured. But if the stress is applied over several days at an optimal rate—not too much but just the right amount for you—then the fitness change becomes measurable. You can produce more power, ride faster, and manage greater levels of stress.

It should be obvious that if you can handle more stress now than you could a month ago, then you are fitter. For now, just for the purpose of understanding the basics of workload, let's examine stress in terms of only one of its components: volume. We'll omit intensity for now. Let's say, for example, that this week you rode for a total of 16 hours, and that was just barely manageable, meaning you were tired but not totally wasted by the end of the week. But a month ago you could cope with only 12 hours as that put you at your limit. Based on this change, I think you would agree that you are in better shape than you were a month ago. Your fitness has improved. If a month from now your weekly volume is 20 hours and it doesn't wipe you out, then you are, once again, seeing an improvement in fitness. So how much stress you can handle over a period of time such as a week is an indirect indicator of fitness. It's indirect in that we aren't measuring any physiological fitness markers, such as VO_2max. Nevertheless, this is a good sign that something positive is happening.

Keep in mind that in the example I used here I was talking only about volume. Intensity, the most important training component, was not factored in. If we can figure out a way to do that, then this whole concept of accumulated stress takes on an even greater level of importance. Let's take a look at how that that can be done with something called the "Training Stress Score."

TSS is merely a way of mathematically combining the duration and intensity of a single workout to produce a number, or "score." This score is more indicative of the stress experienced in a workout than if we talked only about how long or how hard you rode as separate bits of information.

By combining them, we have only one number representing each workout, which allows us to easily compare workouts in terms of how hard or easy they were. Here's how that's done.

Every workout has a TSS. Some power meter head units and analysis software compute this score for you after each ride. The TSS is determined using your ride's duration in seconds, Normalized Power, Intensity Factor, and Functional Threshold Power. The formula used to determine the TSS of a workout comes once again from Dr. Andrew Coggan's seminal work in this area:

(workout duration in seconds × NP × IF) ÷ (FTP × 3,600) × 100 = TSS

The number 3,600 is how many seconds there are in hour, which, you'll recall, is what FTP is based on and remains a constant in the formula. Also, 100 is a constant and is simply there to give us a two- or three-digit TSS.

You'll recognize NP, IF, and FTP as our old friends from previous chapters. They are all measures of intensity—the most important element of training for the experienced athlete. With this concept of TSS, they have even more to do with fitness than as originally explained. In fact, using them in this formula is going to help you measure fitness and fatigue trends while producing peak form on the precise days of your most important races. This is amazing stuff, which I'll get to shortly. First, however, it's important to become comfortable with the idea of TSS as an indicator of workload for a workout and a period of time such as a week.

Let's dig a little deeper into TSS by using an example. On Tuesday you do a workout that is exactly 2 hours (7,200 seconds) long. On checking your head unit after the ride, you see that your NP was 188 watts. You know your FTP to be 250 watts from previous testing, so the IF was 0.75 (188 ÷ 250 = 0.75). If we plug all of these numbers into the TSS formula above, we get

$$(7,200 \times 188 \times 0.75) \div (250 \times 3,600) \times 100 = 112.8$$

Your TSS for this ride was 112.8. We don't know based on this number exactly what type of workout it was and therefore exactly what type of fitness it produced. Your ride could have been a muscular endurance, an anaerobic endurance, or some other ability-type session, as explained in Chapter 4. But we know it was somewhat hard since you rode at 75 percent of your FTP for 2 hours. That's a pretty challenging ride. Once you've established a history of workout scores, you'll soon begin to see patterns. So let's do that for a week.

Your 112.8 TSS for this ride was on Tuesday, we'll say. For every ride this week, you also have a workout TSS. By the end of the week, your daily TSS might look like this in your training log:

Monday	0 (day off)
Tuesday	112.8
Wednesday	80.5
Thursday	100.6
Friday	72.8
Saturday	101.2
Sunday	153.9

Each daily TSS was calculated using the above formula. This gives us some idea of how hard your rides were. We can see, for example, that Tuesday, Thursday, Saturday, and Sunday were the hardest rides, as shown by relatively high TSS. Monday, Wednesday, and Friday were apparently recovery days. The most difficult ride was on Sunday.

If we add all of these daily scores, we get a weekly workload of 621.8 TSS. So now we have what we never had before—a way of expressing how challenging a week was by using *both* volume and intensity instead of volume only. As we said earlier, increases in workload mean an increase in fitness. That is, you become more fit if you train longer and more intensely. Therefore, if 621.8 is greater than what you were capable of doing a month ago, you now have a concrete indication that you are more fit. In putting together the TSS number, we're simply using the training components known to produce a biological phenomenon called fitness to create a mathematical model.

Now it's time to take a look at how you can use TSS to monitor fitness in order to be ready on race day. That has to do with periodization.

POWER AND PERIODIZATION

If you've been around your sport for any time at all, you've undoubtedly come across the concept of periodization. "Periodization" is merely a fancy term for how you organize training relative to time. You can schedule hard and easy days and hard and easy weeks. That's a basic way of periodizing in order to stress your body and yet also allow time for recovery so that you do not wind up overtrained. The TSS calculation sharpens this concept. In fact, through the use of TSS, you can precisely manage the level of stress to increase your fitness, limit fatigue, and produce peak performance on race day.

Fitness

What is fitness? As athletes we throw that word around a lot, yet seldom do we stop to consider what it means. In terms of athletic performance, it's simply the state of being ready to race at a high level of performance. Training is therefore specific to a given race. Fitness for a cyclist doing a 1-hour criterium is nothing like the fitness required to race an Ironman triathlon.

So the training for these events will be significantly different even though they both involve riding a bike. The differences will be evident in terms of how long (duration) and how hard (intensity) the workouts are. The TSS scores for a crit rider and an Iron-athlete may be the same for some of their key workouts, but the ways they get to those scores are completely different. One emphasizes high duration and moderate intensity (Ironman); the other focuses on high intensity and moderate duration (criterium).

Both athletes will watch their daily and weekly TSS to make sure they are increasing their fitness. As explained earlier, they'll know if they are making progress because both daily and weekly TSS will increase over time. What was once a hard TSS will eventually become an easy TSS, and so the workouts are gradually made harder to apply stress and therefore make the athlete more race ready.

You can observe that TSS progression using software and a chart called "Performance Management" (WKO+ and TrainingPeaks.com provide this feature). The software assumes, with good reason, that changes in fitness are slow and occur over many days—probably over several weeks, in fact. It may take 6 weeks to actually see measurable indications of improved fitness, such as an increase in VO_2max. The improvement doesn't happen overnight.

With this in mind, what the software does is produce a daily rolling average of your TSS for 6 weeks—42 days. (That's the default setting; you can manually change that setting in the software if you believe you are an exceptionally fast or slow "responder.") The software takes your TSS for today's workout, adds it to the previous 41 daily TSS, divides by 42, and places that average TSS-per-day data point on a chart. You can see such a Performance Management Chart™ in Figure 7.1.

On this chart the X axis is time in days for one entire season, with the first day on the left end being October 21, when the training season started,

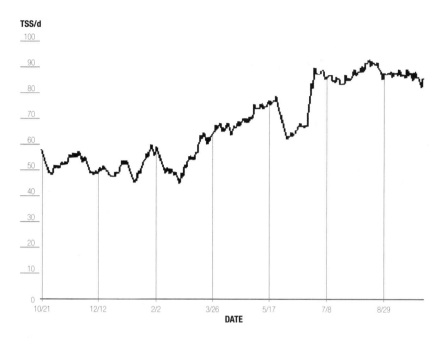

FIGURE 7.1 Performance Management Chart showing chronic training load (fitness)

and the last on the right end being September 1, when it ended. The Y axis is TSS per day (TSS/d). Each daily data point is the 42-day average up to and including that day. The data points have been connected to show how TSS, or fitness, has changed over time. As the line rises, fitness can be assumed to be increasing, also. A dropping line suggests a loss of fitness.

Now realize, again, that I'm using the word "fitness" in a nonspecific way. The line doesn't say anything about "fit for what"—crit or Ironman. It only shows that the athlete is capable of handling more training workload or less, which, as explained earlier, can be used as a proxy for fitness. The software avoids this issue by calling the connected data points the "Chronic Training Load"™ (CTL).

Call it what you want, but what we are seeing here is an increased (or decreased) capacity for training stress management. But having a high CTL, such as 93 in Figure 7.1, doesn't mean that you can outrace your training partner whose CTL at the same point in time is only 76. This number is not reflective of actual performance compared with others. Your CTL at any given time shows only *your* trends—how you are doing now compared with previously.

Having such a tool allows you to manage your training by controlling how fast the line rises or falls. You can watch and control trends using it. When CTL rises, you are undoubtedly becoming more fit because you are coping with more stress. But you are also becoming more fatigued.

Fatigue

You should now understand the relationship between TSS and fitness. As you increase your training workload, as reflected by an increasing CTL on the Performance Management Chart, your fitness improves. Of course, these same increases in TSS per day are also going to make you more fatigued. Greater training workloads make you tired. So if fitness improves with a rise in TSS per day and fatigue also increases as TSS per day rises, then we can draw the conclusion that both fitness and fatigue follow the same trends. In other words, if you train hard, you will become both more fit and more fatigued. If you decrease your training workload, both fitness and fatigue will also decline. That may seem obvious now, but as we get deeper into this, you may question that logic as it applies to race preparation. But stick with me, and I'll show you that the truth of this statement does not contradict your experience.

The Performance Management software calculates daily data points for fatigue in the same manner as was done for fitness (CTL). Only instead of the calculation being based on a 42-day rolling average, it is based on 7 days (again, this is a default setting in the software and may be changed). The reason for this metric is that fatigue occurs and diminishes rather quickly when compared with fitness. The day after a hard ride, you are not able to measure changes in fitness since they are so small, but you can, indeed, sense fatigue. There's no doubt that you're tired. But a day or so later, after some recovery, the fatigue is almost gone. So since this calculation has to do with brief periods of time, the software calls this fatigue the "Acute Training Load"™ (ATL).

CTL and ATL sound very important, but I refer to them instead as fitness and fatigue when I discuss performance management with athletes. While these terms aren't precisely fitness and fatigue in a biological sense, they are good indicators of what's happening in the body and much more easily understood. So for our purposes, CTL = fitness and ATL = fatigue.

Figure 7.2 illustrates the fatigue (ATL) for the same rider whose fitness (CTL) was described in Figure 7.1. Notice how much more "spiky" the rider's fatigue line is than the fitness line for the same period of time. Again, that's because fatigue occurs rather quickly and to a greater magnitude, so a rider is very aware of it in contrast with the slower response of fitness.

By overlaying the rider's fitness (CTL) and fatigue (ATL) lines, we get a clearer picture of what was experienced over the course of the entire season. This is done in Figure 7.3. Whenever the fatigue line is above the fitness line, we know that fatigue is quite high. Notice the huge spike in fatigue in mid- to late June at the same time that fitness is steadily rising. We know from this that the athlete was training very hard during this 2-week period. Fitness was rising, but fatigue was extremely high. That was preceded by a period of no training at all in late May, as can be seen by the rapidly falling fitness and deeply dipping fatigue lines. In fact, this chart describes quite well what was going on with the rider over the course

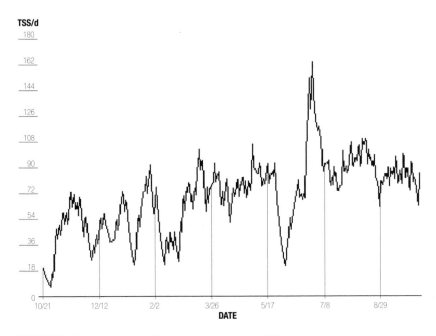

FIGURE 7.2 Performance Management Chart showing acute training load (fatigue)

of an entire season. It's the backdrop for a long story the athlete could tell us about that season. And yet all it represents is data downloaded from the power meter every day.

If you fail to download workout data, then this chart and others are useless. You must be dedicated to doing this for every ride without exception. If there are days that you can't download because of other commitments, don't fret. The head unit stores the data, which can be downloaded later. It is capable of storing several such workouts. How many depends on which head unit you have, how it is set up, and how long the rides were. Consult your user's guide for the details of your device.

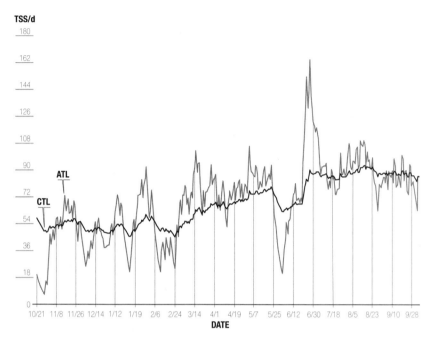

FIGURE 7.3 Performance Management Chart showing CTL (fitness) and ATL (fatigue)

Form

The Performance Management Chart can also be used to help you peak on race day. Peaking, sometimes called "tapering," is a periodization method in which duration is reduced while racelike intensity is maintained. (I explain the process of peaking in greater detail in my books *The Cyclist's Training Bible, The Triathlete's Training Bible*, and *The Mountain Biker's Training Bible.*) The ultimate goal of peaking is to come into "form" on race day. You've undoubtedly heard this term used before by athletes and perhaps by sports commentators on TV. They refer to being "on form." No one ever explains what this means, however, because, I expect, few really understand it. Being on form is not simply possessing high fitness, although that's part of it. I'll explain.

The term "form" is thought to have originated with the popularity of horse racing in Europe in the late 1800s. If you went to the racetrack and wanted to bet on a horse, you would go to a bookie (a betting agent). He would have a sheet of paper with a list of all of the horses in the race, their odds of winning, and a brief summary of how they had been racing recently. You would pick a horse to bet on from this information because it looked good "on the form"—the sheet of paper. This eventually became "on form."

Bike racing, which was coming into prominence at about this same time, adopted this term since there was also betting at these races. It stuck, and so for well over a century cyclists have referred to being on form. In recent years, other sports have adopted the term, so it's used across a broad spectrum of activities from cycling to running to golf and more—including mountain biking and triathlon.

But if on form doesn't mean just being fit, what does it mean in the context of racing? What it really means is that the athlete is race ready. Being race ready indicates that fitness is high and, more importantly, that the athlete is fresh—rested. We already know about fitness, which is CTL on the Performance Management Chart. So how do we measure freshness? We can answer that by better understanding the process of tapering and peaking.

As mentioned earlier, when you taper, you reduce your daily TSS (workload) while including some brief, racelike workouts. Remember from our discussion earlier what happens when you reduce TSS: You lose fitness. Still okay with that? Perhaps not? Most athletes believe that when they taper, they gain fitness. However, you *can't* reduce TSS and gain fitness. It just doesn't work that way. If stress is reduced, fitness begins to fade away. If doing less training were the key to fitness, you would sit in front of the TV to get fitter.

When fitness (CTL) decreases, what happens to fatigue (ATL)? Well, remember that they trend in the same directions, but they do so at different magnitudes. So tapering will also cause a loss of fatigue. That's not a bad thing; cutting fatigue means that you become fresher. And that's the payoff: When you cut back on TSS, you gain freshness—you come into form. You must reduce TSS even though it will also cause a loss of fitness. But that's okay. This conundrum is resolved by the other unique dimension of fitness: It decreases at a slower rate than does fatigue.

If you are careful with your training, you can reduce fatigue a lot over the course of a couple of weeks while decreasing fitness only a little. Time it right and you will be on form by race day. You'll race better if you have given up a lot of fatigue even though you've lost a little fitness along the way. A highly fit but tired athlete doesn't perform as well as slightly less fit but well-rested athlete. Fatigue is more powerful than fitness. It must be eliminated even if that means giving up a little fitness.

Another way of expressing this relationship among fitness (CTL), fatigue (ATL), and form during tapering is to say that we are focused on sub-tracting fatigue. When we think of it this way, the formula for form becomes

$$\text{Fitness (CTL)} - \text{Fatigue (ATL)} = \text{Form}$$

Again, we only want to lose a little fitness while shedding a lot of fatigue in order to come into form. It's a careful balance we're trying to achieve between CTL and ATL. With this balance between CTL and ATL in mind, form is referred to in the Performance Management Chart as "Training Stress Balance" (TSB). That's another fancy term, so I'll continue to call it form except when discussing the numerical data point it represents on the chart.

Figure 7.4 adds form (TSB) to the athlete's fitness (CTL) and fatigue (ATL) from the two previous figures. Every day the TSB data point was determined by the subtraction of the previous day's ATL from that same

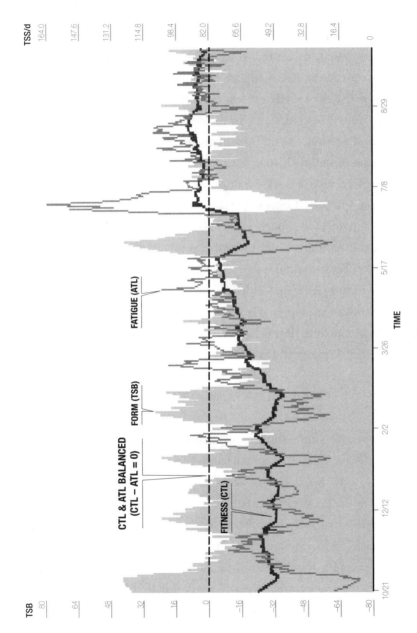

FIGURE 7.4 Performance Management Chart showing CTL (fitness), ATL (fatigue), and TSB (form)

day's CTL. If ATL and CTL are exactly the same, then TSB is 0 and the bars rise to exactly the dashed line across the chart (the zero TSB line). Any time TSB is above that line, meaning a positive number, the athlete is on form. When TSB is rising, the athlete is "coming into form" even though TSB may be below the zero-balance point, meaning a negative number. Coming into form means moving toward being race ready but not being quite there yet. We need to include periodization to keep TSS on track during the taper period, as we'll see next.

PERFORMANCE MANAGEMENT

So where do you want your form—your TSB line—to be? If the TSB line goes too high, you will also lose a great deal of fitness. That's not good. What I like to do is to design the training program for an athlete so that form (TSB) on race day is between +15 and +25. That usually means a loss of CTL (fitness) of only about 10 percent. That's acceptable. If the fitness deficit is much greater, we can expect a significantly diminished performance despite a very high TSB.

To plan for a +15 to +25 TSB on race day, I use the calendar view of the software and put in what I think the TSS should be for every day during the taper period. This period usually lasts 2 to 3 weeks, so it involves estimating TSS for several days. Then I look to see how these estimated daily TSS workloads affected CTL and TSB on the Performance Management Chart. If the result isn't what I want (TSB at +15 to +25 and CTL dropping no more than 10 percent), then I tinker with the daily TSS projections until I get them right. The final step is to design daily workouts to create those TSS and CTL values. It's a somewhat long and laborious task but a highly effective one, I've found. I expect that in the not-too-distant future the software will be able to do much of this for you. But as of this writing, we're not quite there yet.

I EXPECT YOU CAN NOW understand why I explained at the start of this chapter that what was going to be discussed here was quite advanced. This is cutting-edge training. It's the kind of stuff that only a handful of the best coaches in the world do in training their athletes. Very few athletes even know about such planning. And even fewer do it. It isn't easy and certainly takes some time and a good deal of understanding about training. But it can be done by anyone who has a power meter, software (WKO+ or TrainingPeaks.com), and a strong desire to perform at the highest possible level.

PART III

HOW CAN I USE MY POWER METER TO IMPROVE MY COMPETITIVE PERFORMANCE?

8

Power for Road Races and Time Trials

AS A BIKE RACER, you may specialize in sprinting, climbing, or time trialing. Or you may be a multitalented rider who can do quite well in several of these areas for road races, criteriums, time trials, and stage races. The courses you compete on may be hilly, mountainous, or flat. In a road race, the dynamics are constantly changing as riders attack and as little breakaway races occur inside the bigger race. Team dynamics are also at play as your squad decides whether to chase a break, send a rider off the front, set up for a sprint, and so on.

Preparing for such complex racing requires an understanding of what is necessary for success—however you define it—and then carrying out a plan that has you primed and ready to go on race day. This is by no means a simple challenge. Your power meter, coupled with analysis software, makes the preparation much easier. In this chapter I will show you how to use both to race better than you have ever raced before.

WHAT'S IMPORTANT?

If you are new to training with power, then I expect by this point in the book you feel a bit overwhelmed. I've thrown a lot of information about power at you. Before reading this book, you probably never would have imagined that one number on your handlebars could have so many applications. So let's narrow the discussion to what's important for you right now by looking only at the most important topics for road racing and time trialing. I'll also introduce a couple of other topics that will pull together much of what you've already read. The only purpose here is to help you produce better race results using a power meter.

Training to Race

The physiological demands of racing are specific and definable. The purpose of training is to prepare for those demands. The higher your race goals, the more precisely you must define and prepare. This process is made considerably easier if you understand power. It's even easier if you have power files from previous races. By examining the details of those races, you can begin to define their demands and at the same time create targeted goals for your training.

What should you look for when examining past power data from races? Here's a list that will get you started understanding what a certain race is all about, including the chapter in which you can find an in-depth description of that topic.

ROAD RACE ANALYSIS

- Normalized Power and Intensity Factor for the entire race and for key segments such as hills (Chapter 4)
- Matches burned in sprints, out of corners, on hills, in the peloton, and in breakaways (Chapter 5)

- Peak Power for various durations, but especially for 5 minutes or less (Chapter 5)
- Training Stress Score for the race, including warm-up (Chapter 7)
- Training Stress Balance on the day of an A-priority race (Chapter 7)
- Signs of excessive fatigue during the race (Chapter 5)

TIME TRIAL ANALYSIS

- Variability Index for the entire race and for well-defined segments (Chapter 5)
- Intensity Factor for the entire race and for well-defined segments (Chapter 6)
- Training Stress Balance on the day of an A-priority race (Chapter 7)
- Signs of excessive fatigue during the race (Chapter 5)

Let's take a closer look at a few of these topics from the specific point of view of road and time trial racing.

Racing with a Power Meter

The ever-changing nature of a road race forces you to make quick decisions on the fly. Should you go with a break that's forming? Can you close a gap? In a break, should you sit on or work hard? Should you lift the pace on a climb? What should you do if you find yourself off the front solo? Knowing your Peak Power for various durations will help you make such decisions.

First, let's review Peak Power from Chapter 5. That's the highest power you are currently capable of sustaining for a given period of time. Since the outcomes of road races are mostly determined by what happens in brief episodes usually lasting less than 5 minutes, knowing your current Peak Power for such durations helps you make decisions.

Here's an example of how this might work. You're on a climb and about 5 minutes from the top. The small group you're in has been climbing steadily for 10 minutes, and your power has been right around 290 watts. That's close to your FTP, so this is an easily sustained effort. You realize, however, that there are a couple of riders in your small group who are breathing hard. If the pace were to be lifted a bit in the next few minutes, they would probably be dropped. No one else seems willing to make this happen. So you decide to lift the pace and reduce the size of the group. How hard should you go? You happen to know that your Peak Power for 5 minutes (P5) is 360 watts. But with a bit of fatigue in your legs after an hour of racing, that may be difficult to maintain to the top. So you decide to bump your power up another 40 watts to around 330. That will still leave you with a comfortable margin in case another rider matches and raises your effort. So you go.

This decision-making process took only a few seconds. It's typical of what you can do to race smarter by knowing your capabilities in terms of power. But having a power meter on your handlebars will allow you to make decisions only if you know what the numbers mean. That's why you must have power software so that you can analyze workouts and, especially, races. The data you collect has tremendous potential for improving your race results. Let's examine a few more ways it can be beneficial.

Road Race Pacing and Energy Conservation

Pacing is something road cyclists seldom talk about. It's occasionally brought up in discussions of time trial racing but is rare when the topic is a road race or criterium. No one seems to think of these latter two events as demanding any sort of intensity regulation.

How many races have you done in which the field bolted from the start line as if shot from a cannon? That's quite common. I'm sure you've experienced it many times. You may have even been one of the riders at the front who helped lead the charge. There may occasionally be a good reason for a team to do this. Perhaps the strategy is to put pressure on another rider or team right from the gun. But more commonly, I expect, overly fast starts are due to pent-up emotions accompanied by an adrenaline rush. If that's the case, then there is no performance benefit to this kind of start. It only wastes energy and produces an early spike in blood acidosis levels.

Superfast starts are less common as the experience level of the peloton increases. You will seldom see the Pro/I/II field charge away from the start line of a road race, but helter-skelter starts are the norm in Category IV races. Experienced riders understand the importance of conserving energy for when it is really needed. There is nothing to be gained in the first 2 minutes of the race, but a lot can be lost. You have no control over how fast others ride from the get-go—and you have to be ready to go with them—but you can sit in and not be one of the jackrabbits.

If you want to contend for a podium position or even just improve on your race results, the key is to race using the least amount of power possible. The ultimate Normalized Power for a road race or criterium is something as close to zero as you can produce while still competing. In hard workouts you want high numbers on your power meter in order to boost fitness. But in a race the goal is low numbers. Road racing is about conserving energy. That's called pacing. Race smart, not hard.

Figure 8.1 shows a great example of a rider who was smart during a road race. In this cadence-distribution chart, the zero cadence bar on the left side of the chart shows that he coasted for nearly 12 percent of the race. Figure 8.2 shows the resulting power distribution during the same race. Note that for more than 40 percent of the race he was in power zone 1. Staying out of the wind and coasting so much not only reduced the power he used but

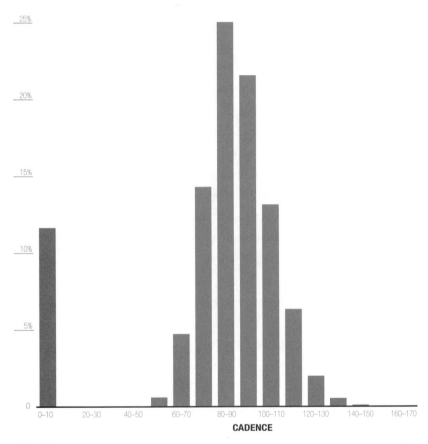

FIGURE 8.1 Cadence distribution from a road race showing that nearly 12 percent of the race was spent coasting at zero RPM

also increased the chances that he would have the energy necessary to climb well, break away from the peloton, or sprint at the finish line. It's no wonder he podiumed in this race. This is a skill you can hone in group rides and C-priority races. In the build period these are your best opportunities to practice patience and control.

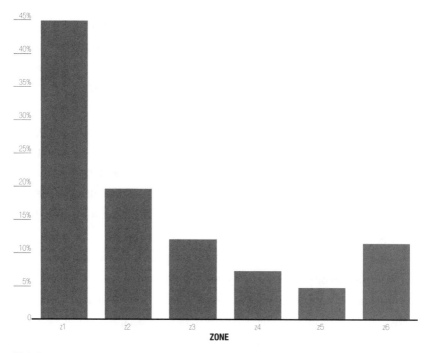

FIGURE 8.2 Power distribution from a road race showing that more than 40 percent of the race was done in power zone 1

Time Trial Pacing and Energy Conservation

In a time trial, pacing is critical, of course. But just as in road racing, the least experienced riders start at much too high an intensity and attempt to maintain their world-record speed for as long as possible. Less than halfway into the race, they are already slowing down significantly. By the last quarter of the race, they are sitting up and wishing it were over. Their hyperenthusiasm coupled with a lack of planning results in a poor performance every time. They will eventually learn how to pace. With a power meter on board, you already know how.

In a time trial the general pacing strategy has been known by racers for decades: When the course is slow, ride hard; when the course is fast, ride easy. That's essentially the 50-40-30-20-10 Rule described in Chapter 5 (Table 5.2, page 83). When the course is slow (uphill) and you are going about 10 kph, work very hard. How hard? Go back to Chapter 5 and reread how to control burning matches on hills in steady-state races (Table 5.3, page 88). When the course is fast and you are going downhill at more than 50 kph, conserve energy by pedaling easier or even tucking and coasting.

Your ultimate goal in a time trial is a fast time. That means starting at a high power just long enough to get up to race speed and then immediately settling in to your planned power. If you paced it right, you will cross the finish line just as you are running out of gas. One of the best indicators of how well you paced a time trial is the Variability Index you see in the post-race analysis. If this is about 1.05 or less, then you paced quite well. If it's above that, you need to practice regulating your effort.

Of course, the VI of a road race or criterium will be much higher and is not a good indicator of how well you raced. That falls into the realm of match burning, which we'll review next.

Proper race pacing boils down to emotion control and patience. Those are easy to come by in a workout, but your greatest challenge is in a race. The more often you race, the better you will get at both. Until smart race pacing becomes second nature, however, it's imperative that you constantly remind yourself before the start to conserve energy.

Key Workouts

Key workouts are the most important ones in your training each week and have the greatest influence on your race readiness. Each consists of a unique and purposeful combination of intensity and duration. Generally, as the duration of a key workout is reduced, its intensity increases. For example, rides in power zone 2 may last for several hours, while burning matches in zone 7 lasts only a few seconds for each match. The type of race for which you are training and its specific demands are the primary determiners for your key workouts.

Early in the season, during the base period, key workouts are the same whether your focus is a road race or a time trial. Your purpose is to boost general fitness. The base period key workouts are primarily intended to improve aerobic endurance and muscular endurance. (Speed skills and muscular force abilities are of secondary importance at this point.) This combination of workouts should elevate your FTP two or more times before the end of the base period. All of this is described in detail in Chapter 6.

In the last 12 weeks or so prior to your A-priority race, the focus of the workouts shifts toward race-specific training with the intent of getting faster. The key workouts now take on the characteristics of the targeted race. Road racers will focus on anaerobic endurance, while time trialists will take their muscular endurance to a much higher level.

In the build period, at least one workout each week must have a Training Stress Score similar to what you expect in the race. If you have a power file for that event from a previous year, you've got a great indication of what the workout TSS should be. If you don't have that power file, ask your training partners who have power meters and who raced in it last year if they would be willing to share their power files. If that doesn't work, at least find out how long the race was and what the terrain was like. From the race length and course profile, and from what you've learned so far about power, estimate the race TSS. That will get you started doing race-simulation workouts.

The purpose of this race-simulation workout is to gradually adapt to the race TSS so that on race day you are well prepared. You may recall that TSS is the product of both duration and intensity, with a slight weighting in favor of intensity. For this racelike workout, TSS is mostly duration based early in the build period but shifts toward more emphasis on intensity as the training period progresses. The workout stays about the same, while the way in which you produce it varies. Let's look at an example of how that may be done.

The targeted event is a road race that last year took 2 hours and 3 minutes to complete. That day you rode for 30 minutes prior to the start to warm up, and so by the end of the race you had accumulated roughly 2.5 hours of saddle time. The race is on a hilly course with a few climbs that ultimately select the riders who will contend for the podium. Last year you were in a small chase group behind three riders who got away on the final climb. You finished second in your group in a sprint at the line, which put you fifth overall and less than 1 minute behind the winner. This year your goal is to make the podium. If your fitness is high and everything goes right, you may even win it.

In reviewing last year's power file, you find your race TSS was 152 with an Intensity Factor of 0.863 (see Chapter 5 for more on IF). Including the warm-up, your total TSS for the day was 177. Given your FTP of 290 watts, your Normalized Power for the race was 250 watts (290 × 0.863). You burned 17 matches, with the longest being 75 seconds and the average duration being 30 seconds. The average match intensity was 369 watts (127 percent of your FTP). The biggest match that day was 475 watts (164 percent of FTP) for 28 seconds. You now have an excellent idea of what the demands of your race were last year, and you can make rather accurate predictions of what is needed this time around. And so you know what you must train to do.

In the build period, you will do a race-simulation workout once a week that focuses on achieving or exceeding the metrics described above. Your club has a 2-hour group ride on Saturdays, which will work perfectly for this key workout. At the beginning of the build period, for the first of these rides, you warm up for 30 minutes by riding to the bike shop where it starts. During the first ride, you do a bit of work at the front, but mostly you sit on to get used to the intensity of a fast-moving peloton. By the end of the group ride, including the warm-up, your head unit tells you that you have a TSS of 132 and an Intensity Factor of 0.727. Your goal for this weekly ride is to exceed 177 (last year's combined race and warm-up TSS), and you eventually want the IF to be well over 0.800. So you put in another 45 minutes after the club ride on your own doing anaerobic endurance intervals. Your total TSS for this 3:15 ride winds up being 186, with an IF of 0.757. That's a good start.

In each subsequent week, you ride a bit more intensely in the Saturday group ride, with an increasing emphasis on riding aggressively on the hills, and you finish each ride with racelike intervals. As a result of the increase in Intensity Factor, even though the total workout duration is getting shorter, the workout's weekly TSS stays about the same—somewhat north of 177. That means the ride is becoming more racelike. By late in the build period, it is nearly as challenging as you expect to see in the race.

What you did throughout the build period was to shift the source of the key workout TSS from duration to intensity. The intensity portions were specifically intended to mimic what is expected in the race. You also did some C-priority races in these final 12 weeks in place of the club ride to gauge your progress and mentally prepare for your A-priority event. By race day you are ready to rock.

Regardless of the type of race for which you are preparing, this concept of simulating the demands of the event—TSS and Intensity Factor—will help you prepare in a way that greatly increases your chances of achieving a high race goal.

Anaerobic Endurance Workouts

In Chapter 5 I told you about match burning in events such as road races and criteriums. This is essentially what such races are all about. Their outcomes are nearly always the result of brief episodes in which Peak Power was very high. Match burning falls into the training-ability category of anaerobic endurance and is another type of key workout in the build period. Such training not only improves anaerobic endurance for racing but also elevates your aerobic capacity (VO_2max). That basically means a bigger engine to power your bike.

Given this latter benefit, I suggest that time trialists also do some anaerobic endurance training. Since most roadies do road races and time trials, even though both may not be A-priority, there is some similarity in the training for both types of events. The only thing that varies is the emphasis. Riders training for a road race also do muscular endurance in the build period—just not as much as a time trial specialist does. And the time trialist also does anaerobic endurance workouts—just not as much as the road racer does.

In order to perform well in a road race, you must be capable of going deeply anaerobic frequently and recovering from these brief episodes quickly. In the build period, if your A-priority race is a road race or crit, then preparing to burn matches should make up a significant part of your training. These are the primary key workouts described below in "Road Race Build Period."

Examples of anaerobic endurance workouts are in Appendix A.

Muscular Endurance Workouts

The purpose of muscular endurance training is to improve your capacity for maintaining an intensity that is near your lactate threshold for a relatively long time. The lactate threshold is roughly the equivalent of your Functional Threshold Power.

Muscular endurance is the most basic of the advanced abilities. For the road racer, it means riding along with no discomfort in a fast-moving group while having plenty of energy in reserve to accelerate and burn a match when the situation calls for it. Muscular endurance is also called on in a road race during a long, solo breakaway. Such workouts are of secondary importance for the road racer. For the time trial specialist, muscular endurance is at the core of race preparation in the build period.

While the key race-simulation workout in the build period for a road racer is anaerobic endurance, for the time trialist it is muscular endurance. If you specialize in time trialing, then this workout must focus on long intervals done at around FTP. Time trials that take about 1 hour mean racing right at FTP. Shorter time trials require a higher Intensity Factor. Races that take longer than 1 hour are done at below FTP. Of course, you must also realize that even though your average Intensity Factor for the time trial may be at or below FTP (an IF of 1.0 or less), there may well be times in the race when you are above FTP. This takes us back to the 50-40-30-20-10 Rule mentioned earlier.

Again, muscular endurance workouts are done by both time trial specialists and road racers. All that varies is the amount of such training done each week in the build period.

Secondary Workouts

Secondary workouts are the sessions that are somewhat less important to your race preparation than are key workouts. If you look ahead to Tables 8.2 and 8.5, you'll see that the training abilities I've included in this category are speed skills (in 8.2), aerobic endurance, and sprint power (in 8.5). Note that aerobic endurance in the early base period is a key workout. After that, your training of this ability should go into a maintenance mode. That's why it's listed in the late base and build periods as a secondary workout.

Being of secondary importance, these workouts may be omitted or modified in some way to better fit your unique needs. For example, if your weekly training schedule must be changed owing to other commitments or situations, such as work or family responsibilities or even threatening weather, these workouts may be left out so that you can fit in the key workouts for the week. Those should always have the higher priority.

Of course, it may also be that a training ability I have classified as secondary in these tables may be of primary concern to you. If you are a sprint specialist, then sprint power sessions could well be key workouts. Or should your speed skills or aerobic endurance be especially poor, there may well be a personal need to elevate one of them to a higher priority.

It's not possible to design a general training plan for everyone who rides and races. Ultimately, you must decide for yourself how your periodization and priorities are arranged. Take what you see in the remainder of this chapter as suggestions. Total program design is outside the scope of this book and is discussed in greater detail in *The Cyclist's Training Bible*.

Recovery Workouts

Periodic recovery is critical to training quality. For an experienced cyclist, this means going for a short and easy spin. Novices are better advised, however, to take a day completely off from training to rejuvenate.

It's common for type-A, experienced riders to do too few recovery rides and too many key workouts. This mistake will ultimately result in some sort of breakdown. Either the body or the mind will soon say "enough" and force you to the couch for an extended time.

Instead of succumbing to exhaustion, you should incorporate active recovery sessions into your training schedule. Don't think of these sessions as wasted time. Riding in zone 1 when fatigued is an effective way for advanced athletes to rejuvenate the body while also maintaining pedaling economy by keeping the cadence comfortably high. You may even consider doing speed skills training during a recovery ride, as most are not too stressful (see Appendix A for examples of speed skills workouts). A recovery ride, however, must be truly easy. Your Normalized Power should be around 50 percent of your FTP by the end of such a ride.

On a recovery day your body needs to adapt to the stresses you've been applying and be allowed to grow stronger. Your body is also replacing expended glycogen stores if the preceding key workout was a high Training Stress Score. All of this takes time and can't be rushed. Your body doesn't care when the next race is or how eager you are to get in shape. It requires recovery.

The biggest mistake many riders make is doing their recovery rides at an Intensity Factor that is well above zone 1, thinking this will produce higher fitness. It won't. It only prolongs the fatigue and reduces the quality of the next key workout. When what should have been a zone 1 recovery ride is done in zones 2 and 3, residual fatigue will linger into the next key workout. That eventually produces a steady diet of mediocre training sessions and an erosion of race performance. The harder your key workouts are, the easier your recovery rides must be.

For the riders I've coached over the years, I've seen that their weekly average Intensity Factor is usually around 0.70 throughout their entire seasons. That's mid–zone 2 and not especially high. It comes from balancing the key and recovery workouts every week. In the base period, a lot of moderately hard rides are done to boost general fitness; they are balanced out with somewhat easy recovery rides. This produces an IF of about 0.70. If a very hard ride with an exceptionally high TSS is done in the build period, it is balanced out by a very easy ride or even a day off (zero TSS). Again, this produces a moderate IF of around 0.70. If your weekly average IF is consistently well above that, perhaps 0.80 or more, you may be on the road to overtraining. You need to either recover more or check your FTP to see if it is perhaps too low. Should your weekly IF be consistently quite low, around 0.60 or less, then either you are undertraining or your FTP is set higher than it should be.

PREPARING FOR YOUR RACE

Chapter 6 introduced the concept of periodization of training, with the base period focused on general fitness and the subsequent build period aimed at getting faster with race-specific training. With your new and deeper understanding of the complexities of power-based training, it's time to get down to the nitty-gritty: preparing to race. We'll look at this topic primarily as an overview of periodization, with a somewhat greater emphasis on the details of workout power. Again, for a more thorough discussion of the periodization of training for cycling, see my book *The Cyclist's Training Bible*.

For this discussion I'm going to assume that you are an advanced athlete. What follows is not intended for novices. A novice is someone in his or her first year of serious training for bike racing. Athletes in their second year in the sport who have been riding about 10 or more hours weekly for at least the previous 12 weeks and nearly all racers entering their third year in the sport are generally ready to move on to advanced training as explained in the following sections. The newer you are to serious cycling, however, the more conservative and cautious you should be with what I'm about to explain.

If you are a novice, the primary focus of your training must be aerobic endurance. This ability is described in detail in Chapter 6, along with power-based tools for measuring the progress of this ability. Muscular endurance workouts, as described below, should be done somewhat conservatively. The novice should include many speed skills workouts and perhaps limited muscular force training (see Appendix A for details on all of these). As a novice, be very careful when training muscular force. This workout is excellent for developing the force component of power (recall from Chapter 1 that power is the result of force and cadence), but it places great stress on the joints, especially the knees. Stop the workout at the first sign of joint discomfort. If your knees are tender, either the workout is too stressful for your current level of fitness, you've been training too hard, or you need a bike fit.

What is primarily described below is intensity, not volume. Volume varies greatly from one athlete to the next. Your purpose in training is not to log a large amount of duration-based TSS every week. It's not how long the rides were but what you did in them to produce the intensity that matters most. As a road cyclist, your focus must be on intensity first, workout duration second, and weekly volume a distant third. Intensity—and duration to a lesser extent—is much more closely linked to your race success than is weekly volume. In what follows there are only brief mentions of duration and no mention of volume regarding racelike training.

Warm-up before the higher-intensity portions of workouts is assumed. The more intense the ride is, the longer the warm-up should be. It doesn't take much warming up for a zone 2 aerobic endurance ride. Ten minutes or so is usually adequate. But prior to zone 5 anaerobic endurance intervals, you need a long warm-up. This could take 20 to 30 minutes of gradually increasing intensity.

TABLE 8.1 BASE PERIOD WORKOUTS FOR THE ADVANCED ROAD RACER AND TIME TRIALIST

PERIOD	KEY WORKOUTS	SECONDARY WORKOUTS
EARLY BASE PERIOD (6–8 WEEKS)	AEROBIC ENDURANCE (AEROBIC THRESHOLD) MUSCULAR FORCE (FORCE REPS)	SPEED SKILLS (DRILLS)
LATE BASE PERIOD (4–6 WEEKS)	MUSCULAR ENDURANCE (SWEET SPOT)	AEROBIC ENDURANCE (AEROBIC THRESHOLD) SPRINT POWER (JUMPS)

See Appendix A for workout details.

This discussion of workouts is divided by periodization into two sections—the base period for all racers and separate sections on the build period for road racers and for time trial specialists.

Base Period (for All Races)

The types of workouts I suggest for the base period are the same for both road racers and time trialists. General fitness, which is your base period goal, is similar across the board for disciplines. The base period workouts are shown in Table 8.1 by training ability, with workout name in parentheses.

In the early base period, the advanced athlete's most common need is the reestablishment of aerobic endurance. This ability may well have declined after a transition period, especially an extensive one that followed the completion of the previous season. If the transition period break from hard and focused training occurs at midseason following an early A-priority race, then you may not need another early base period; your aerobic endurance may not have declined significantly. Treating this ability as a secondary priority in either late base or build period training will more than likely suffice in this situation.

The duration of the aerobic endurance ride for the advanced rider is typically between 2 and 3 hours. But in a maintenance mode it may be half that long. As described in Appendix A, you warm up and then ride steadily in the lower portion of heart rate zone 2 for the duration (use my heart rate zone system as described in Appendix B to make sure the intensity is right). After the ride, when you analyze your workout graph, pay special attention to your decoupling and Efficiency Factor for the zone 2 portion (see Chapter 6 for details). What you want to know is how your power responded to that particular heart rate.

This aerobic threshold workout is the only one you'll do during the season that uses heart rate to gauge intensity. The reason we use heart rate for this workout is that some research has shown that heart rate is likely to decrease as fatigue sets in. That decrease would give us a false impression of improving fitness if you used power as the steady-state, intensity gauge. Power has never been shown to increase with fatigue.

What should you do during this workout if power is obviously decreasing while heart rate remains the same? That's decoupling as described in Chapter 6 and tells you that your aerobic endurance is inadequate. Or you may simply be having a bad day. That happens to everyone from time to time. You may also have had too much caffeine prior to the ride, which could be elevating your heart rate. Anything that affects heart rate could be the culprit. Unfortunately, training is not a perfect world. Press ahead with the workout despite the apparent decoupling. No harm will come from this, and there is still a training benefit.

During this steady ride, there are bound to be interruptions as a result of traffic, stoplights, flat tires, and more. When these occur, just get back to zone 2 as soon as you can and continue on. Over several weeks, assuming the conditions and the courses for this workout don't change radically, minor variations will cancel out as you compare decoupling and Efficiency Factor results over several weeks to gauge aerobic endurance progress.

Speed skills training can be done within another workout since the TSS value isn't very challenging. It can be included in any other rides during the week as drills during warm-up, between reps, or during cooldown.

The most intense key session in the early base period for the advanced rider is muscular force. Limit this workout to only once per week because of its high risk for injury. As always, the first time you do this workout in the base period, start with a low number of repetitions. Over the next several weeks, gradually add more reps as your body adapts. Be conservative and cautious as you progress with this workout. It's risky.

It will probably take you 6 to 8 weeks to optimize your muscular force. A good sign that you are ready to move on is that your Peak Power for 6 seconds (P0.1) in this workout will stabilize. When you see this happen, it's time to substitute muscular endurance training for the muscular force workouts.

The muscular endurance workout of the late base period is quite simple, involving only 2 intervals of 20 minutes each done at 88 to 93 percent of FTP with a 5-minute recovery between them. That's high zone 3 to low zone 4 power. Dr. Andrew Coggan, the guru of training with power, calls this power range the "sweet spot." It's a very effective and efficient workout for increasing FTP. An additional 4 to 6 weeks of such training should bring your general fitness to a high level.

A typical week of workouts in the early and late base periods for an advanced cyclist may look something like the examples in Tables 8.2 and 8.3. There are many ways to arrange your workouts in the base period. These are but two examples.

TABLE 8.2 SUGGESTED WEEKLY, EARLY BASE PERIOD WORKOUTS FOR THE ADVANCED ROAD RACER AND TIME TRIALIST

DAY	WORKOUT
MONDAY	(DAY OFF FROM TRAINING)
TUESDAY	AEROBIC ENDURANCE
WEDNESDAY	RECOVERY (ZONE 1)
THURSDAY	MUSCULAR FORCE + SPEED SKILLS
FRIDAY	RECOVERY (ZONE 1)
SATURDAY	AEROBIC ENDURANCE
SUNDAY	MUSCULAR FORCE + SPEED SKILLS

See Appendix A for workout details.

TABLE 8.3 SUGGESTED WEEKLY, LATE BASE PERIOD WORKOUTS FOR THE ADVANCED ROAD RACER AND TIME TRIALIST

DAY	WORKOUT
MONDAY	(DAY OFF FROM TRAINING)
TUESDAY	AEROBIC ENDURANCE
WEDNESDAY	MUSCULAR ENDURANCE
THURSDAY	RECOVERY (ZONE 1)
FRIDAY	SPRINT POWER + AEROBIC ENDURANCE
SATURDAY	RECOVERY (ZONE 1)
SUNDAY	MUSCULAR ENDURANCE

See Appendix A for workout details.

Road Race Build Period

Since most cyclists do both road races and time trials, even though the training emphasis may vary in the build period, the key and secondary workouts are the same. Table 8.4 lists those workouts.

TABLE 8.4 BUILD PERIOD KEY WORKOUTS FOR THE ADVANCED ROAD RACER AND TIME TRIALIST

PERIOD	KEY WORKOUTS	SECONDARY WORKOUTS
BUILD PERIOD (8–9 WEEKS)	MUSCULAR ENDURANCE (CRUISE INTERVALS) ANAEROBIC ENDURANCE (FAST GROUP RIDE, VO₂MAX INTERVALS, MATCH-BURNING INTERVALS) SPRINT POWER (JUMPS, HILL SPRINTS)	AEROBIC ENDURANCE (AEROBIC PACING) SPRINT POWER (JUMPS, HILL SPRINTS)

See Appendix A for workout details.

As a road racer, your most important training goal in the build period is to increase the number of matches you can burn, increase how long you can burn them, and increase the Peak Power of the matches. As explained under the "Key Workouts" section earlier, the starting point for such training is to go back to race files you have stored on your computer or online, especially for the A-priority race for which you are currently training, and search for matches burned (the sidebar in Chapter 5, "How to Set Up WKO+ for Matches," page 86, tells you how to do this with WKO+ software). You can define a match any way you want. I use power in excess of zone 6 (Table 4.1, page 63) for more than 20 seconds in a road race and 10 seconds for criteriums. You could also define them differently—for example, say a match is zone 6 or higher for 1 minute or more. Regardless of how you set them, search for your matches burned in the previous year's race file. Armed with this information, you are now able to create workouts that mimic the demands of the race to help you prepare to burn more matches, longer matches, and bigger matches.

You also need to continue developing muscular endurance. This should have come along quite well in the late base period as indicated by an increased FTP when you come to about 12 weeks before your race. Now, if you do cruise intervals as explained in Appendix A, these workouts will become more challenging and your FTP is likely to rise again.

TABLE 8.5 SUGGESTED WEEKLY BUILD PERIOD TRAINING ABILITIES FOR THE ADVANCED ROAD RACER

DAY	WORKOUT
MONDAY	(DAY OFF FROM TRAINING)
TUESDAY	ANAEROBIC ENDURANCE
WEDNESDAY	RECOVERY (ZONE 1)
THURSDAY	MUSCULAR ENDURANCE + SPRINT POWER
FRIDAY	RECOVERY (ZONE 1)
SATURDAY	RACE SIMULATION + ANAEROBIC ENDURANCE
SUNDAY	AEROBIC ENDURANCE

See Appendix A for workout details.

You should also maintain aerobic endurance in the build period by doing such a workout once a week. Table 8.5 suggests this for Sunday, the day after your racelike key workout. Generally, riders are fit enough at this point in their training that such doubling up is not an issue. And, in fact, with a proposed day off the bike on Monday, the workload is usually manageable. But if you find you are too wasted on Sunday to ride even in zone 2, you may need to rearrange things to better fit your recovery status.

Time Trial Build Period

Table 8.4 lays out the suggested build period workouts for both the time trial specialist and the road racer. While the categories of workouts are similar for the two disciplines, the emphasis varies. With a focus on the time trial, your main emphasis must be on muscular endurance. That's your core ability. The other primary ability is anaerobic endurance, but your type of training is significantly different from that of the road race specialist for this session. Unless you're also doing B- or A-priority road races, you're less concerned with burning matches. Your focus for the anaerobic endurance workouts is on building a greater aerobic capacity (VO_2max), as this will translate into faster time trials.

Of secondary importance in your build period training are aerobic endurance and sprint power. The aerobic endurance workouts are intended to maintain the gains made in this category during the base period. One long ride per week, done in zone 2, will accomplish this. Unless you are also doing road races, you may omit the sprint power session. This is an optional workout and if included can be on any day in the week that best fits your needs.

Table 8.6 provides a suggested weekly build period training plan for the time trialist. The most important workouts here are Tuesday and Saturday. The Saturday race-simulation ride is best done on a course that is similar to the one on which you will be racing. This calls for doing intervals at your race Intensity Factor with an emphasis on increasing the duration of each interval or on decreasing the time of the recoveries between them. Be sure to apply the 50-40-30-20-10 Rule and match burning for steady-state races on hills (see Chapter 5 for details on both of these).

The per-hour TSS for the Saturday ride is likely to be around 55 to 60, and it will probably take 2 hours or less. If so, I'd suggest adding a steady, aerobic endurance ride after the intervals to bring the total workout TSS up to about 150. If you do that, then ride for recovery on Sunday. But if you end the Saturday ride after the intervals, do a long, steady, aerobic-pacing ride in power zone 2 on Sunday. Make this the 150-TSS day instead.

Road Race and Time Trial Peaking

The last 2 to 3 weeks before your A-priority race is the time to start coming into form for the race. You do this by making some changes to your training load. Chapter 7 explains the details of Chronic Training Load, Acute Training Load, and Training Stress Balance. It may be helpful at this point to go back to that chapter and reread the section "Power and Periodization" to refresh your memory on the details of coming into form.

TABLE 8.6 SUGGESTED WEEKLY BUILD PERIOD TRAINING ABILITIES FOR THE ADVANCED TIME TRIALIST

DAY	WORKOUT
MONDAY	(DAY OFF FROM TRAINING)
TUESDAY	MUSCULAR ENDURANCE
WEDNESDAY	RECOVERY (ZONE 1)
THURSDAY	ANAEROBIC ENDURANCE (+ SPRINT POWER)
FRIDAY	RECOVERY (ZONE 1)
SATURDAY	RACE SIMULATION (+ AEROBIC ENDURANCE)
SUNDAY	AEROBIC ENDURANCE (RECOVERY)

See Appendix A for workout details.

The bottom line for the peak period—the final 2 or 3 weeks before your most important races—is raising your TSB (form) by reducing ATL (fatigue). You do this by gradually reducing your daily and weekly TSS for this 2- to 3-week period of time. You may remember that reducing workout TSS, which is done primarily by reducing workout duration (not intensity), results in the loss of a little bit of fitness and in a lot of fatigue. Consequently, form rises. Using WKO+ software or its online equivalent, TrainingPeaks.com, you can manage and even predict what your TSB (form) will be on race day.

What you're after on race day is what I call "strong form." That means CTL (fitness) has decreased only about 10 percent or less from the start of the peak period 2 to 3 weeks out from your race, and TSB (form) has risen into the range of +15 to +25. "Weak form" may still produce an in-range TSB, although it's usually much too high, but fitness will drop by more than 10 percent. Back in Chapter 7, I described how you can manage and predict your race-day CTL and TSB by plugging in TSS numbers that you forecast for every day in the upcoming 2- to 3-week peak period. If the Performance Management Chart shows that CTL and TSB are not where you want them to be on race day, then you simply jigger the projected daily TSS numbers around until CTL and TSB are correct.

What I've found works quite well for this tapering process is to do a racelike workout every third day during the peak period. The IF must be quite close to what you expect to happen on race day. These workouts must be quite hard. But they get shorter every time you do one, meaning their TSS and the week's cumulative TSS will decline throughout the peak period.

Between these racelike key workouts, you do recovery rides. They must be zone 1 and also may get shorter as the peak period progresses. Plug estimated TSS numbers for each key and each recovery workout throughout the peak period into your WKO+ or TrainingPeaks.com calendar, and you will create a specific plan of action to be on form on race day. Then you simply need to do the right types of workouts on those days in order to produce the projected TSS. It's simply amazing how we can now use power and analysis software to do something that used to be all guesswork and hoping.

BICYCLE RACING IS A COMPLEX SPORT and is as much an art as a science. Race preparation requires that you first become generally fit and then translate that fitness into being fast for racing. All of this is inextricably tied to a given day when the race is scheduled. Being ready to race at a peak level on that day has always been a guessing game, with the most critical component being how intensely you should train. Now, with a power meter on your bike and analysis software on your computer, the guesswork is gone. Preparing to race has become more science based and precise.

9

Power for Triathlons

GORDO BYRN, A TRIATHLON COACH and former pro triathlete who specialized in the Ironman distance, once told me that he recalled the happy days of the early 2000s when he was the only pro in the race with a power meter. While everyone else was guessing how to manage intensity on the bike, Gordo would simply race to a wattage number for which he had trained and hold it, with slight variations, throughout the race. He did very well, clocking a personal best of 8:29 at Ironman Canada and winning Ultraman Hawaii using a power meter.

While you may not be that fast or race as a pro, I have no doubt that using a power meter in your training and racing will also give you a leg up on your competition. Those racing and training with only a heart rate monitor are at a definite disadvantage. In this chapter I will show you how to use your power meter specifically for triathlon.

WHAT'S IMPORTANT?

So far in this book you've read about many ways to train using a power meter. Not all of what you've read is necessarily applicable to your preparation for a triathlon. Here I'd like to emphasize the most important points and introduce other triathlon-related topics that will help you make the best use of your power meter in order to race faster.

Training Time

Perhaps the greatest challenge facing you as a triathlete is making the best use of your limited training time. The fewer hours you have for training each week, the greater is the challenge—and the more important your power meter becomes.

Novices typically do 1 workout per day with 2 swims, 2 rides, and 2 runs in a week. That's not much, but at that level they still progress even with what may appear quite limited training. A steady routine of only 6 weekly sessions, however, does not work for the more advanced triathlete. Two workouts per sport in 7 days would soon cause a drop in fitness and race readiness. As the level of accomplishment in the sport rises, so does the volume of training necessary to continually improve fitness. The same holds true as the distance an athlete is preparing to race gets longer. An Ironman requires much more training than does a sprint triathlon.

Even if you have an abundance of time, the mere nature of a three-pronged sport means that time must somehow be distributed in such a way as to optimize your race readiness. How much time will you devote to each sport? The starting point for answering this question is determining how much time you spend in each of the three sports during a race. For most triathletes, that roughly works out to something like 15 percent swimming, 50 percent cycling, and 35 percent running. Your percentages may be slightly different, but you can use these numbers as a starting point for deciding how much time to train weekly in each sport. Then make adjustments to accommodate strong and weak sports. For example, if you are a strong cyclist who has lots of room for improvement in running, shifting some training time from bike to run is probably a good idea.

The bike will still make up close to 50 percent of your race time, so cycling should more than likely be the sport to which you devote the most time. I've seen only a few athletes who were so strong in cycling and so weak in another sport that they needed to ride very little. This is rare. More than likely you ride a lot, as you should. Your power meter will get lots of use and will largely determine how well you do on race day.

Pacing and Intensity Factor

If the bike is the key to triathlon success, the way to race well is to become as bike fit and fast as possible and then hold back when riding in a race so that you have fairly fresh legs for running. I can't emphasize this last point enough: You must learn to hold back slightly during the bike leg of a triathlon. If you come out of T2 thoroughly wasted, then your run will be poor, if you can call what you're doing at that point "running." Walking is more likely. The time you may have "gained" on the bike will be lost—plus more— on the run due to excessive fatigue.

Pacing on the bike at the proper Intensity Factor (see Chapter 5 for more on IF) is critical to your finishing time. If you don't pace well, you don't race well. The swim can, and often does, start with a sprint, which may last for several minutes as the faster swimmers thin the field. By the time the run leg starts, fatigue and reality are starting to take their toll, and so starting the run too fast out of T2 is unlikely. That leaves the bike. It's the one leg that must be well paced. That, again, means holding back, especially at the start. I've seen Ironman triathletes set a personal best time for the first 25 miles of the 112-mile bike leg. And you know what happens after that: The remainder of the day is a slow and painful attempt to finish.

As a triathlete, you must become extremely disciplined when it comes to pacing, and you must incorporate this discipline into your training. Every key workout you do in the build period must be paced at your race-appropriate Intensity Factor so that you finish strongly. For example, in the first interval of a set, restrain yourself by controlling your emotions and the tendency to go very hard. Hold back. Save your hardest effort for the last interval. Try to make that one the best.

When simulating race Intensity Factor, slightly hold back in the first quarter of the ride in order to have a strong final quarter. Closely managed pacing must become habitual so that when you're in a race, it's second nature to hold back. I drill this into every triathlete I coach. Although this restraint is critical to success, self-coached triathletes seldom take it seriously. Intensity Factor and pacing using a power meter are explained in great detail in Chapter 5.

Smart pacing also implies always striving for a low Variability Index as also described in Chapter 5. VI should almost always be 1.05 or lower in a triathlon. A higher VI tells you that you were sloppy with pacing and that you wasted a great deal of energy. Check VI after your race to ensure your steadiness in pacing throughout the entire race, not just at the start. Your overall race time will be faster if you do.

In Chapter 5 I also told you about the 50-40-30-20-10 Rule and provided Table 5.3 (page 88) showing how to control your matches burned by modifying steady-state race power when going up hills. Both of these pacing strategies need to be rehearsed in workouts as well. If you don't practice these pacing skills in training, you are unlikely to do them on race day.

In the final analysis, the key to successful triathlon racing is restrained and steady bike pacing at the appropriate Intensity Factor. Get this right, and you will have a good race.

Racing with a Power Meter

What a miraculous tool the power meter is. You should always race with it. It will help you to properly race the bike leg, and the data you collect will demonstrate what you must do to improve. You will not make the best use of power if you only train with it and never use it in a race.

Unfortunately, many triathletes don't race with their power meters. For example, the popular PowerTap system uses meters built into the hub of the rear wheel, so most triathletes have a training wheel built up with a Power-Tap but race on another rear wheel that's lighter and faster. That means there is no power data during the race. The result: These athletes can't manage intensity or analyze how they did in order to improve next time.

One way to overcome this dilemma is to have two PowerTap wheels—one for training and one for racing. Yes, I hear you: That's very expensive and therefore not a great option. A better solution is to simply buy a nice race wheel with a PowerTap built into it and then use it for training as well. (I'd recommend clincher tire race wheels; clinchers are less expensive when you have a flat, and the speed and handling differences between clinchers and tubulars are now small.) Wheels these days are quite light and yet very durable. A good, dual-purpose wheel will last several years even if you are a high-mileage rider. I've had athletes put in more than 10,000 training miles a year on their "race" wheels and have them last for several years without a problem. You'll undoubtedly want new wheels in three to five years anyway; technology is always changing for the better. And it's psychologically easier to replace a well-used wheel than one that has been mostly hanging in your garage for several years. So if you're going the PowerTap route, get one good rear wheel and use it for all your training and racing.

Bike Selection

It's not unusual for a triathlete to have two bikes: one triathlon-specific bike and one road bike. Triathlon bikes are perfect for flat to gently rolling courses, but when you've got a hilly race coming up, it may be a good idea to use your road bike with clip-on aero bars.

Switching between bikes often means changes in power. You may find that your FTP on a triathlon bike is lower than on your road bike. This is due to differences in position. The more aggressive your aero position (primarily meaning a low front end), the less power you can produce. That may seem counterproductive, but it's a good trade-off. Giving up a few watts on your tri bike while greatly decreasing the drag that holds you back at high speeds on relatively flat terrain means faster times. Road bikes, however, are better for climbing hills, where drag is inconsequential but gravity must be overcome. Sitting upright and back on the saddle allows you to engage the pedal earlier in the downstroke, thus producing more power and climbing faster.

All of this means that you may need two sets of power zones since your FTP could differ depending on which bike you're on. If you anticipate racing at some point on your road bike, check your FTP on it sometime in the base period to see if it is different from that of your tri bike. If the difference is less than 3 percent, there's no need to make any changes to your zones. It's simply not enough to be concerned with. One set of zones will do for both bikes. But greater differences require a unique set of zones for each bike.

This discussion also means that you may find your FTP has changed slightly following a bike fit, which you should have at least annually. If after a fitting session your bike position was changed a great deal—either more or less aggressive—you should retest to see if your zones have changed. Do this right away; don't wait until your next race.

Key Workouts

Key workouts are the ones that have the greatest impact on your race readiness. They involve some unique combination of intensity and duration. Generally, the shorter the duration, the higher the intensity. Rides in power zone 2 may last for several hours, while intervals in zone 6 are only a few minutes each. The race distance for which you are training is the primary determiner for your types of key workouts.

With three sports and so many workouts to do, you'll probably find you can fit in only 1 to 3 key bike sessions in a week. The number depends on several factors, such as how generally fit you are, how well you recover, what period of training you're in, how strong you are on the bike compared with the swim and run, and available training time. The fewer key bike workouts you do in a week, the more important it is to focus on aerobic endurance and muscular endurance in the base period and racelike rides in the build period.

If you can do only 1 or 2 key bike sessions in a week, "combined" workouts are a very effective use of your time. These are workouts that combine two or more training purposes into a single workout. They are most commonly done in the build period. There are many ways to create a combined workout. For example, you could combine muscular endurance intervals and a steady aerobic endurance ride into a single session. Or you could even combine three abilities by, for example, adding anaerobic endurance intervals to the other two.

While combined workouts have great potential for you as a triathlete, do not make them so challenging that you struggle to finish and then spend several days recovering. The progression of a certain type of combined workout needs to be conservative, with the highest level of the total TSS for a session increasing gradually over several weeks. To do otherwise is to risk excessive fatigue, burnout, injury, and illness.

Appendix A provides the details for workouts by ability, but it doesn't offer suggestions for combining them. There's a little bit of science and art involved in creating such a workout. The science part is easier to explain.

Determine the demands of the race, and compare them with your strengths and weaknesses. You have a "limiter" wherever your weaknesses overlap with the race's demands, and a limiter will decrease your chances of having a good performance. For example, a common limiter for the bike is climbing hills. That's a weakness for many triathletes. So if you have a hilly race coming up and hills are a limiter, then you need to build hill training into your combined workouts. Early in the build period, do the limiter portion within the combined workout first. For the example described above, you could do the muscular endurance intervals on a hill followed by the aerobic endurance portion on flat terrain. Late in the build period, work on your limiter in the latter part of the combined workout. In the example, this would mean doing the aerobic endurance ride first, followed by the muscular endurance hill intervals.

The other portion of a combined workout generally focuses on your strengths. Let's say that's pacing. In that case, early in the build period you'd do something such as muscular endurance intervals on a hill (limiter) followed by a long, steady pacing segment at race power (strength). Late in the build, you'd reverse these—pacing first and hills second. Of course, there are many, many other possibilities for limiters and strengths. So, in a nutshell, that's the *science* of combined-workout design.

The *art* of designing combined workouts has to do with analyzing the subtle nuances of your current state of race readiness and then making decisions about what is needed. The possibilities are endless and beyond the scope of this book. I explain them in greater detail in my book *The Triathlete's Training Bible*.

Recovery Rides

Recovery is critical for serious triathletes. I'm afraid many, if not most, hard-charging triathletes simply don't do enough easy workouts. Active recovery sessions in zone 1 have been shown to be an effective way for advanced athletes to rejuvenate the body when tired. For novices, however, a day completely off from training is far better.

Running is not a good option when it comes to active recovery. It's just too stressful for the legs. Swimming is good for such recovery, but it can be difficult to fit into your day when you have to travel any distance to the pool or when facilities are limited. The bike is usually an excellent option for a serious triathlete's recovery day. But a recovery ride must be truly easy. Stay in power zone 1 while riding steadily. Your NP should be around 50 percent of your FTP by the end of the ride. The biggest mistake triathletes tend to make is to do these recovery rides at too great an intensity because they believe that this approach will result in greater fitness. It won't. It will only leave you a bit too tired to have a high-quality session during your next key workout. When what should have been a zone 1 recovery ride is done at a moderate intensity, such as zone 3, you'll carry a bit of additional fatigue into the next key workout and you'll have a mediocre session. A steady diet of moderate-intensity "recovery" rides eventually will cause an erosion of race performance. The harder your key workout rides, the easier your recovery rides should be. When someone tells me he or she isn't racing to potential, the intensity of recovery rides is the first thing I ask about.

Training Partners

Triathlon is an individual sport. Riding with groups during training sessions is often counterproductive because such workouts can deteriorate into miniraces. And even when they don't, you will likely be riding at either too great or too low a wattage for your purpose, whether that purpose is aerobic endurance, muscular endurance, or racelike power. You're also likely to develop bad pacing habits, decrease fitness, and generally not get what you need from the ride.

For the triathlete, the worst groups to ride with are groups of roadies. You may think that such rides are good for your fitness and race preparation since your heart rate and power will peak at high levels several times, accompanied by labored breathing. You'll probably see new seasonal highs for P1 and P6. While that's good for your training partners' purpose in getting ready for variably paced road races, it isn't beneficial to you. Short, spiked bursts of power don't translate into faster triathlon racing. There's little to be gained. These rides may be fun, but they are usually a waste of your precious training time.

A good time to ride with training partners is when you want to recover, but only if the other riders are of similar ability and agree to ride at a controlled effort. It is even better if everyone has a power meter and similar FTPs. You can agree to ride at an Intensity Factor of less than 60 percent, for example (see Chapter 5 for details on IF).

PREPARING FOR YOUR TRIATHLON

Now I want to take you through the four common triathlon distances and describe general training and key workouts for each by period. For a more thorough discussion of the periodization of training for triathlon, see my book *The Triathlete's Training Bible*.

For this discussion, I'm going to assume that you are an advanced tri-athlete, not a novice. I'll define a novice as someone in the first year of tri-athlon training who does *not* have a background in cycling. Triathletes in their second year in the sport who have been riding about 5 or more hours weekly for the previous 12 weeks, and nearly all triathletes entering their third year in the sport, are generally ready to move on to advanced train-ing as explained below. The newer you are to serious cycling, however, the more conservative and cautious you should be with what I'm about to explain.

If you are a novice, your primary focus, regardless of race distance, is aerobic endurance. This ability is described in great detail in Chapter 6, along with power-based tools for measuring its progress. Muscular endur-ance workouts, as described below, should be done somewhat conservatively. The novice triathlete should include many speed skills workouts, largely in the form of pedaling drills, and perhaps limited muscular force training (see Appendix A for details on all of these). Novices must be very careful when training for improved muscular force. It places great stress on the joints, especially the knees, and should be done with caution. Always stop the work-out at the first sign of something that doesn't feel quite right. Never continue a workout when there is joint discomfort. If you feel knee tenderness, the workout is either too stressful for your current level of fitness, you've been training too hard, or you need a bike fit.

The key workouts described below are the workouts most likely to help the advanced athlete improve fitness and become faster. They should be the focus of your bike training every week. If you must miss a ride during a given week of training because of other commitments, try to skip something other than a key session. This usually means rearranging your workouts in a week so that recovery isn't compromised.

Note that the descriptions of the key workouts below are intentionally brief. You will find greater detail in Appendix A.

Note, too, that what we are primarily focused on below is intensity, not volume. Volume varies greatly among athletes. As explained earlier, it's safe to assume that the longer the race, the greater the volume of training. (From Chapter 7, recall that volume refers not only to hours but also to Training Stress Score.) This does not mean simply trying to log a large number of hours or a high TSS every week. It's not the number of hours or the size of the TSS that matters most but what you did with them. The training volume for a long-course triathlete is generally greater than that for a short-course triathlete simply because longer races demand longer rides, not just more short rides. In what follows there are only brief mentions of duration in the discussion of racelike training.

Warm-up before the rides described below is assumed. The more intense the ride will be, the longer the warm-up that precedes it should last. It doesn't take much warming up before doing a zone 2 aerobic endurance ride. Ten minutes or so is usually adequate. But you need a long warm-up before taking on zone 5 anaerobic endurance intervals. The warm-up could consist of 20 to 30 minutes of gradually increasing intensity.

This discussion of triathlon workouts is divided by periodization into two sections: the base period for all race distances and the build period by unique race distance.

Base Period

The types of workouts in the base period are the same regardless of race distance. Your base period goal is general fitness, which is similar across the board for all triathlon distances. The base period workouts are shown in Table 9.1 by training ability, with the workout name in parentheses.

TABLE 9.1 BASE PERIOD WORKOUTS FOR THE ADVANCED TRIATHLETE

PERIOD	KEY WORKOUTS	SECONDARY WORKOUTS
EARLY BASE PERIOD (6–8 WEEKS)	AEROBIC ENDURANCE (AEROBIC THRESHOLD) MUSCULAR FORCE (FORCE REPS)	SPEED SKILLS (DRILLS)
LATE BASE PERIOD (4–6 WEEKS)	MUSCULAR ENDURANCE (SWEET SPOT)	AEROBIC ENDURANCE (AEROBIC THRESHOLD)

See Appendix A for workout details.

All that varies in the base period is the duration of the workouts based on the race distance for which you're training. For example, the steady-state, zone 2 portions of the aerobic threshold workouts vary by distance, as shown in Table 9.2. This is the primary key workout for early base period triathlon training. As described in Appendix A, you warm up and then ride steadily in the lower portion of heart rate zone 2 for the duration, as shown in Table 9.2 for your race distance. After the ride, when you analyze your workout graph, pay special attention to your decoupling and Efficiency Factor for the zone 2 portion. What you want to know is how your power responded to that particular heart rate.

This aerobic threshold workout is the only one you'll do during the season that uses heart rate to gauge intensity. The reason we use heart rate for this workout is that some research has shown that heart rate is likely to decrease as fatigue sets in. That decline would give us a false impression of improving fitness if you used power as the steady-state gauge. Power has never been shown to increase with fatigue.

The first aerobic threshold ride you do in your base period should not be the duration shown in Table 9.2. It should be shorter. It may be half or even less of the ultimate duration for which you are striving. Over the course of this 6- to 8-week portion of the base period, continue to lengthen this ride until you settle in at the goal duration.

What should you do during this workout if power is obviously decreasing while heart rate remains the same? That's decoupling (as described in Chapter 6), and it tells you that your aerobic endurance is not where it must ultimately be. Or you may simply be having a bad day, which happens to everyone from time to time. You may have also had too much caffeine prior to the ride. Anything that affects heart rate could be the culprit. Unfortunately, training is not a perfect world. Press ahead with the workout despite the apparent decoupling. No harm will come from this, and there is still a training benefit.

During this steady ride, there are bound to be interruptions due to traffic, stoplights, flat tires, and more. When these occur, just get back to zone 2 as soon as you can and continue on. Over several weeks, assuming the conditions and courses for this workout don't change radically, minor variations will cancel out as you compare decoupling and Efficiency Factor results over time.

The durations of the muscular force, speed skills, and muscular endurance workouts are the same across the board regardless of race distance.

TABLE 9.2 THE DURATION OF THE ZONE 2, STEADY-STATE, AEROBIC ENDURANCE WORKOUT BY RACE DISTANCE

TRIATHLON RACE DISTANCE	AEROBIC THRESHOLD WORKOUT DURATION*
SPRINT	60 MINUTES
OLYMPIC	90 MINUTES
HALF-IRONMAN	150 MINUTES
IRONMAN	240 MINUTES

* Does not include warm-up and cooldown.

Speed skills training can be done within another workout since the TSS value isn't very challenging. Speed skills can be included in any other rides during the week as drills during warm-up, between reps, or during the cooldown.

The most intense key session in the early base period for the advanced athlete is muscular force. Limit this workout to only once per week because of its high risk for injury. As always, start with a low number of repetitions the first time you do this workout in the base period. Over the next several weeks, gradually add more reps as your body adapts. Be conservative and cautious as you progress with this workout. It's risky.

It will probably take you 6 to 8 weeks to fully develop muscular force. A good sign that you are ready to move on is that your Peak Power for 6 seconds (P0.1) will stabilize. When you see this happen, it's time to substitute muscular endurance training for the muscular force workouts.

The muscular endurance workout of the late base period is quite simple, involving only 2 intervals of 20 minutes each done at 88 to 93 percent of FTP with a 5-minute recovery between them. That's high zone 3 to low zone 4 power. Dr. Andrew Coggan, the guru of training with power, calls this the "sweet spot." It's a very effective and efficient workout for increasing FTP. An additional 4 to 6 weeks of such training should bring your general fitness to a high level.

A typical week of key workouts in the base period for an advanced triathlete may look something like the example in Table 9.3. Remember, these are only the key workouts; you'll certainly have more swims and runs to do as nonkey workouts. You may also need to add additional rides intended for recovery only. How many of these additional workouts you add depends on your unique characteristics as an athlete. Moreover, there are many ways to arrange your key workouts in the base period. This is but one example.

TABLE 9.3 BASE PERIOD KEY WORKOUTS FOR THE ADVANCED SPRINT-DISTANCE TRIATHLETE

DAY	KEY WORKOUT
MONDAY	(DAY OFF FROM TRAINING)
TUESDAY	RUN KEY WORKOUT
WEDNESDAY	BIKE FORCE REPS + SPEED SKILLS (EARLY BASE) BIKE SWEET SPOT + SPEED SKILLS (LATE BASE)
THURSDAY	SWIM KEY WORKOUT
FRIDAY	(ACTIVE RECOVERY RIDE, ZONE 1)
SATURDAY	RUN KEY WORKOUT
SUNDAY	BIKE AEROBIC THRESHOLD

See Appendix A for workout details.

Build Period

Once your base period training is complete, you are ready to move on to the key bike workouts for your build period. The key workouts in the build period vary according to the type of triathlon you are preparing for. Here are the key bike workouts for each of the common triathlon distances. (See *The Triathlete's Training Bible* for a more thorough discussion of training in all three sports.)

Sprint build period. Sprints have the greatest variability in terms of the bike distance of any of the common triathlons. The bike portion is generally in the neighborhood of 10 to 15 miles and may take an advanced triathlete 25 to 45 minutes to complete. If this were a stand-alone bike time trial, it undoubtedly would be raced in power zone 5. Such an effort would create a lot of acidosis accompanied by heavy breathing and burning legs. But since you have to come off the bike and run 5 km or so, you must hold back (here I go again with the "hold back" thing!). With this in mind, you will probably be riding in the range of high power zone 4 to low power zone 5 depending on the duration of the bike leg. The longer the duration, the lower the intensity.

TABLE 9.4	BUILD PERIOD KEY WORKOUTS FOR THE ADVANCED SPRINT-DISTANCE TRIATHLETE	
PERIOD	**KEY WORKOUTS**	**SECONDARY WORKOUTS**
BUILD PERIOD (8–9 WEEKS)	MUSCULAR ENDURANCE (CRUISE INTERVALS) ANAEROBIC ENDURANCE (VO$_2$MAX INTERVALS)	AEROBIC ENDURANCE (AEROBIC THRESHOLD)

See Appendix A for workout details.

Table 9.4 shows the key and secondary workouts for the advanced, sprint-distance triathlete during the build period.

The key workouts for the advanced sprint-distance racer's build period are muscular endurance (cruise intervals) and anaerobic endurance (VO$_2$max intervals). If the bike portion of your race will take more than 40 minutes, then place greater emphasis on the former. In fact, that may be the only key workout in your build period if your bike split will be greater than 45 minutes. But if your race is quite short, less than 30 minutes, then stress anaerobic endurance.

One of your weekly rides in the build period should simulate the intensity and duration of your race. This will need to be done as intervals—either cruise intervals or VO$_2$max intervals, depending on your anticipated bike duration. Always finish this race-simulation ride with a short run of 5 to 10 minutes at race intensity.

You should also maintain aerobic endurance in the build period by adding a 30- to 60-minute portion done in zone 2 to one of your other key rides once each week to make a combined workout. For this workout especially, but for all workouts generally, be sure to manage your pacing by following the 50-40-30-20-10 Rule and managing your match burning (Table 5.3, page 88). This is a critical component for becoming not only fitter but also faster.

TABLE 9.5 SUGGESTED WEEKLY BUILD PERIOD KEY WORKOUTS FOR THE ADVANCED SPRINT-DISTANCE TRIATHLETE

DAY	KEY WORKOUT
MONDAY	(DAY OFF FROM TRAINING)
TUESDAY	RUN KEY WORKOUT
WEDNESDAY	BIKE VO₂MAX INTERVALS (OR CRUISE INTERVALS)
THURSDAY	SWIM KEY WORKOUT
FRIDAY	(ACTIVE RECOVERY RIDE, ZONE 1)
SATURDAY	RUN KEY WORKOUT
SUNDAY	BIKE RACE-INTENSITY SIMULATION + AEROBIC THRESHOLD (+ T2 RUN)

See Appendix A for workout details.

Table 9.5 provides an example of a build period training week for an advanced sprint-distance triathlete.

Olympic build period. At 40 km, the bike leg of an Olympic-distance triathlon is raced at just below FTP for most athletes. Elites, who may post a bike split of around 50 minutes, will probably race at FTP. That will be "holding back" for them. All others will be riding in the lower portion of zone 4. How low depends on how long the bike portion takes. Those who produce a time of about 70 to 80 minutes should ride at the very low end. If your time is projected to be in the range of 60 to 70 minutes, then your power should be close to but slightly below your FTP. Of course, as with all training and racing, it's critical that your FTP is currently accurate.

The emphasis for Olympic-distance training is primarily on muscular endurance in the build period. While the elite with a sub-1-hour bike split may want to include some anaerobic endurance training in the form of

TABLE 9.6 BUILD PERIOD KEY WORKOUTS FOR THE ADVANCED OLYMPIC-DISTANCE TRIATHLETE

PERIOD	KEY WORKOUTS	SECONDARY WORKOUTS
BUILD PERIOD (8–9 WEEKS)	MUSCULAR ENDURANCE (CRUISE INTERVALS)	AEROBIC ENDURANCE (AEROBIC THRESHOLD)

See Appendix A for workout details.

VO_2max intervals, this is not recommended for those who will finish in more than 1 hour. The potential reward doesn't offset the risk for such athletes.

The key workouts for the advanced Olympic-distance triathlete are shown in Table 9.6.

Once each week in the build period, include a race-simulation workout. For the advanced rider at this distance, that means doing cruise intervals, as described in Appendix A. At the start of the build, about 12 weeks out from the race, do intervals on the shorter end of the recommended range, such as 5 to 6 minutes. That would produce a cumulative interval time of 25 to 30 minutes. Over the next 8 weeks, gradually increase the interval durations. By about 3 weeks before the goal race, you should be doing in the range of 40 to 60 minutes of cumulative interval time. For example, that may be 5 intervals of 8 minutes each (40 minutes total) or 5 intervals of 12 minutes each (60 minutes total).

If you will be racing on a hilly bike course, consider doing your race-simulation cruise intervals as repeats on a hill that is similar to what you expect on race day. That will probably mean your recoveries are longer than 25 percent of interval duration. That's okay. Just get back down the hill, and start the next interval as soon as possible.

For your weekly race-simulation workout, transition to a short run following the bike ride. About 10 to 15 minutes of running at race pace is all that's

TABLE 9.7 SUGGESTED WEEKLY BUILD PERIOD KEY WORKOUTS FOR THE ADVANCED OLYMPIC-DISTANCE TRIATHLETE

DAY	KEY WORKOUT
MONDAY	(DAY OFF FROM TRAINING)
TUESDAY	RUN KEY WORKOUT
WEDNESDAY	BIKE CRUISE INTERVALS
THURSDAY	SWIM KEY WORKOUT
FRIDAY	(ACTIVE RECOVERY RIDE, ZONE 1)
SATURDAY	RUN KEY WORKOUT
SUNDAY	BIKE RACE-INTENSITY AND DURATION SIMULATION + AEROBIC THRESHOLD (+ T2 RUN)

See Appendix A for workout details.

needed. The purpose here is not to build fitness but to become comfortable at transitioning from the bike to a race-intensity run. This is part of what I mean about becoming faster, not necessarily fitter, in the build period.

During the build period, it's also important to maintain aerobic endurance. An hour or so of aerobic threshold riding at the low end of your heart rate zone 2 once a week will do this. It could be a stand-alone workout or tacked on after an interval session. It is *not* a recovery workout.

Table 9.7 provides an example of how you may arrange your key workouts in the build period.

Half-Ironman build period. Also often referred to as the 70.3 distance or even as a "long-course" triathlon, a half-Ironman-distance race should more accurately be thought of as a "double-Olympic-distance" race. That's because the demands of such a distance are closer to those of the shorter race than to those of the longer. For the fastest half-Ironman triathletes, the training is also similar to what an Olympic-distance racer does.

TABLE 9.8 BUILD PERIOD KEY BIKE WORKOUTS FOR THE ADVANCED HALF-IRONMAN-DISTANCE TRIATHLETE

PERIOD	KEY WORKOUTS	SECONDARY WORKOUTS
BUILD PERIOD (8–9 WEEKS)	MUSCULAR ENDURANCE (CRUISE INTERVALS AND/OR TEMPO INTERVALS)	AEROBIC ENDURANCE (TEMPO INTERVALS)

See Appendix A for workout details.

Those who will split the bike in about 2 to 2.5 hours should do cruise intervals, as described in the Olympic-distance discussion earlier. That means 30 to 60 minutes of interval time done at power zone 4 in 1 workout weekly. The long ride is a race-simulation session with tempo intervals in zone 3.

For those who expect their bike leg to be completed in more than 2.5 hours, the only key bike workout is tempo intervals. This is both the single-purpose weekly ride and the longer race-simulation ride.

Tempo intervals are 20 minutes long and done in power zone 3 with 5-minute recoveries in power zone 1. See Appendix A for details. Zone 3 is more than likely the intensity you will race at for this distance. Faster triathletes will race in upper zone 3 to lower zone 4 (Intensity Factor 0.85 to 0.95). All others will be in mid– to low zone 3 (Intensity Factor 0.75 to 0.85). Training and experience will help you narrow the IF to a much smaller range. Your key workouts as suggested below should reflect this expected Intensity Factor.

Table 9.9 suggests 2 key bike rides in a week. One of them may include only 2 or 3 tempo intervals (for example, the Wednesday key workout in Table 9.9), while the other (Sunday in Table 9.9) will top out at 6 intervals about 3 weeks prior to race day. Progress gradually to 6 over the course of the build period. Start the build period with 2 or 3, and work your way up. The longer session (Sunday in Table 9.9) is your race-simulation workout, so finish it with a short run of 15 to 20 minutes at race pace.

TABLE 9.9 SUGGESTED WEEKLY BUILD PERIOD KEY WORKOUTS FOR THE ADVANCED HALF-IRONMAN-DISTANCE TRIATHLETE

DAY	KEY WORKOUT
MONDAY	(DAY OFF FROM TRAINING)
TUESDAY	RUN KEY WORKOUT
WEDNESDAY	BIKE TEMPO OR CRUISE INTERVALS
THURSDAY	SWIM KEY WORKOUT
FRIDAY	(ACTIVE RECOVERY RIDE, ZONE 1)
SATURDAY	RUN KEY WORKOUT
SUNDAY	BIKE RACE-INTENSITY AND DURATION SIMULATION + AEROBIC THRESHOLD (+ T2 RUN)

See Appendix A for workout details.

Tempo intervals will maintain your aerobic endurance, so there is no reason for the half-Ironman triathlete to do zone 2 rides in the build period.

Ironman build period. The bike leg of the Ironman is, without doubt, the key to race success. If you want to run well, you must achieve top bike fitness and then hold back during the race. Typically, an Ironman bike leg is generally raced in the IF range of 0.65 to 0.75. Most age-group triathletes will race between 0.65 and 0.70. Only the elites finishing in well under 5 hours will be close to 0.75.

At the start of the bike leg on race day, this IF will feel amazingly easy, and your inclination will be to disregard your power strategy and go faster. Adding to your sudden decision to abandon the pacing plan will be the many, many riders passing you in the first 5 miles. If you dump your pacing plan now and go with them, you'll regret it in the last quarter of the bike leg and all during the marathon, which you will likely be walking. Once you have an effective IF for the race, stick with it. Be patient. Those passing you early in the race will come back to you later.

TABLE 9.10 BUILD PERIOD KEY BIKE WORKOUTS FOR THE ADVANCED IRONMAN-DISTANCE TRIATHLETE

PERIOD	KEY WORKOUTS	SECONDARY WORKOUTS
BUILD PERIOD (8–9 WEEKS)	MUSCULAR ENDURANCE (TEMPO INTERVALS) OR AEROBIC ENDURANCE (AEROBIC PACING)	AEROBIC ENDURANCE (AEROBIC PACING) OR MUSCULAR ENDURANCE (TEMPO INTERVALS)

See Appendix A for workout details.

Considering all of the common triathlon race distances, Ironman is the one in which your power must be most closely monitored and controlled since the race is so long. Your race-day Variability Index, the 50-40-30-20-10 Rule, and match-burning control are critical to success. All training rides must incorporate these markers of effective pacing.

For the advanced Ironman triathlete, there are 2 key bike workouts in the build, as shown in Table 9.10.

The shorter and more intense session (Wednesday in Table 9.11) consists of tempo intervals, as described in Appendix A. You are most likely to use this intensity in the race on hills. So do this session as repeats on a hill, if possible. If there are no hills where you live, then you have no choice but to do the tempo intervals on flat terrain. That's not optimal, but there's no other option.

The other key bike workout is aerobic pacing. The only difference between this and the aerobic threshold workout you did in the base period is that now you are using power instead of heart rate to gauge intensity. Our purpose is no longer to simply develop aerobic endurance but rather to rehearse and refine a pacing strategy for race day. During the build period, you should come to know exactly what your Intensity Factor must be for the race and how you will vary it to adjust for hills.

For professionals, many of the athletes will start the race at an IF closer to 0.80 in order to maintain contact with the lead group. There are several advantages, both psychological and aerodynamic, to being with this group at the pro level. But the intensity of these few pros will slowly drift downward as the bike portion of the race progresses. By the end of the race, most will be closer to an IF of 0.70. They must train for such a pacing strategy.

For the age-group triathlete, this is a disastrous way to race. There is no need to stay with a lead group since there are likely to be athletes nearby throughout the race. You must develop a pacing strategy based on an IF that keeps you just fresh enough to run at a decent pace. That's the purpose of long-day training (Sunday in Table 9.11) during the build period.

In addition to pacing, the other critical component of your Ironman success is on-bike eating. Ironman is a swim-bike-run-and-eat contest. If you don't adequately replace expended carbohydrate stores during the race, you are unlikely to be able to run or even to finish. The key is to match race IF with caloric intake rates. The higher your IF, the lower the amount of

TABLE 9.11 BUILD PERIOD KEY WORKOUTS FOR THE ADVANCED IRONMAN-DISTANCE TRIATHLETE

DAY	KEY WORKOUT
MONDAY	(DAY OFF FROM TRAINING)
TUESDAY	RUN KEY WORKOUT
WEDNESDAY	BIKE TEMPO INTERVALS
THURSDAY	SWIM KEY WORKOUT
FRIDAY	(ACTIVE RECOVERY RIDE, ZONE 1)
SATURDAY	RUN KEY WORKOUT
SUNDAY	BIKE RACE-INTENSITY AND DURATION SIMULATION (+ T2 RUN)

See Appendix A for workout details.

food you can process and the more likely it will be a liquid. As IF gets lower (meaning a slower finishing time), caloric intake can increase and food can become more solid. Long rides in the build period are the only ways of figuring all of this out. They must be done at the proper IF while you experiment with refueling options (see my book *The Paleo Diet for Athletes* for more details on this).

TRIATHLON IS A COMPLEX SPORT. Getting the proper mix of swimming, biking, and running wedged into your life is certainly a challenge. Your power meter can help with all of this by enabling you to practice in training what is critical for your success in racing. At the most basic level, that means paying special attention to Intensity Factor and pacing. Training with power takes these critical ingredients to your success from guesswork to precision. Training and racing with a power meter are almost like cheating. And they're easy once you get the hang of them.

10

Power for Century Rides

RIDING 100 MILES IS A DAUNTING TASK, even if your only goal is to finish. It is an even greater challenge if you've set your sights on achieving a personal best time for the century. That's when a power meter really shines. In this chapter I'll show you how to apply what you've read in previous chapters to have your best century ever. You'll delve more deeply into the key workouts that will help you become fitter and faster. And I'll suggest weekly training plans that will bring you right up to the day of your century in top form. This is going to be fun. Let's get started.

WHAT'S IMPORTANT?

In the first seven chapters, I may have overwhelmed you with information on power. You may now feel that training for your century using a power meter is a complicated process—perhaps even beyond what you think is possible. I can assure you that it isn't. The key to preparation is to focus on the most important parts of your century preparation and on how a power meter can make your training better.

Effort and Intensity Factor

To have a good century ride, you must get two things right: Intensity Factor and Variability Index. Both are described in Chapter 5. Let's review Intensity Factor first to see why it is so critical.

You probably recall that Intensity Factor measures the effort of your ride. It's found by dividing the Normalized Power for a ride by your Functional Threshold Power. An IF of 1.0 indicates that your NP and FTP for that ride were exactly the same. In other words, you completed the ride at your FTP. That would be one tough ride, however, since by definition FTP is the highest power you can produce for 1 hour. Riding 1 hour at redline is beyond the ability of most riders.

In fact, there's absolutely no way you're going to complete your century ride with an IF of 1.0 or even close to that. For most participants, the fastest century rides take about 5 hours, putting their IF in the range of 0.75 to 0.8. That's a hard ride for 5 hours. Riders at the other end of the spectrum, finishing in 7 hours or longer, will have an IF around 0.5 to 0.6. Most will ride at an IF of 0.6 to 0.7.

So, in general, we can safely say that most riders in a century will have an IF between 0.5 and 0.8. That translates into the high end of power zone 1, power zone 2, and the low end of power zone 3. One of your goals in preparing for the century is to figure out what your "base" IF should be. This is the IF you'll maintain on relatively flat terrain. You can determine it by looking at past century ride files to see what your IF was. If you don't have any such files, start paying close attention to your IF on long rides. You'll probably ride with a bit of greater effort in the century, but the training rides will give you a general indication of what to expect.

Once you know your anticipated IF, you must learn to do your long rides at about that effort. Don't wait until the day of your century to do this. It's too late by then.

The other important piece for having a successful century ride is pacing, especially when you aren't on flat terrain at your base IF. We'll look at that next.

Pacing and Variability Index

Pacing is critical to your performance in a century. This has much to do with how efficiently you use energy, especially your precious glycogen stores. Glycogen is the carbohydrate-based fuel your body will use, along with fat, to provide fuel to turn the cranks. There's some mix of the two fuel sources being used throughout the ride. Your glycogen supply is limited, however; you may have 1,500 to 2,000 calories of glycogen socked away, mostly in your muscles. If you go hard and fast for a while, you'll burn more glycogen and less fat. If you slow down, the blend of the two fuels will reverse and your body will rely more on fat.

Since you have only a small amount of stored glycogen to draw from but lots of fat (even the skinniest rider has enough fat stored away to ride for a few days), you'll need to take in carbs while riding in the form of sports drinks, bars, gels, or whatever you like to eat and drink. The problem is that your gut can process only a limited amount of such stuff— probably 200 to 350 calories per hour while riding, depending on your body size and a few other variables. If you take in more than your digestive system can process, the carbs (and whatever else you may have consumed) will just sit there, causing a bloating feeling and perhaps nausea. That's not good.

Glycogen is clearly a valuable resource, so it is wise to be very conservative in your expenditure of glycogen during your century to avoid premature fatigue. The way to do this is to manage your IF and strictly limit your surging during the ride. It takes more glycogen to surge than to ride steadily, even if in the end your average power output is the same. Every time you surge, such as when you try to prevent someone from passing you, charge up a hill, or hook up briefly with a fast-moving group, you burn glycogen at a much higher rate. If you do this repeatedly during a century ride, even though you are taking in carbohydrate, you are likely to get behind the fuel output-input curve. In other words, you may start running low on glycogen. If that happens, the party's over. This is called "bonking" and is the greatest challenge facing the serious century rider.

The key to steering clear of the feared bonk is to take in carbs at a known and manageable rate and pace your ride fairly steadily. The first part has to be determined in your training rides. It's largely based on experience—trial and error—as we're all different when it comes to refueling. The second part takes us back to several concepts discussed in Chapter 5 that I think we should review now from your unique perspective of training for a century.

Let's start with the Variability Index. Recall that this feature of the WKO+ software and TrainingPeaks.com tells you how steadily you rode. It's found by dividing Normalized Power by average power. If they are exactly the same, then your VI is 1.0. That means you rode very steadily. If you changed pace frequently, then your VI will increase to something greater than 1.0. For your century ride, and for most of your key workouts, you should aim to keep your VI at around 1.15 or less. If it's well above 1.15 for a century ride, then you are likely wasting a lot of energy.

"But," you may ask, "what if there are hills on the course? Won't that cause me to *not* ride steadily?" Yes indeed, hills will affect your VI. How much depends on how aggressively you ride up the hills. If you surge and slow down repeatedly on a long hill or aggressively attack short ones, your VI will go way up. Instead of that, the idea is to ride up hills at an intensity you can steadily maintain to keep your overall VI in the neighborhood of 1.15 or less. That's the premise of Table 10.1, which you can think of as your match-burning guide for century rides. It suggests that on hills you can increase your power output by up to two zones. For example, since most century rides are done in power zone 2 (IF of 0.55 to 0.75), depending on how fast the rider is, then hills are best climbed in power zone 4. How long you can safely stay in a higher zone and how much cumulative higher-zone riding you can do in a single century are also suggested in Table 10.1. This is only a rough guideline, as some people can handle more and some less. Once again, the only way to learn what you can manage is to rehearse it on your training rides.

That brings us to the 50-40-30-20-10 Rule, also discussed in Chapter 5. As you'll see, it is fundamentally important to your performance. The rule says that when you are riding along at 50 kph (about 30 mph), you're obviously going down a hill. During your century, don't try to go faster. Instead, conserve energy (that precious glycogen) by getting as aerodynamic as you

TABLE 10.1 MATCH SIZE BY ZONE AND DURATION AND CUMULATIVE TIME FOR CENTURY RIDES			
BASE ZONE	ZONE THAT BURNS A MATCH (AND UPPER LIMIT OF INTENSITY)	DURATION IN ZONE THAT BURNS A MATCH (MAY VARY)	RECOMMENDED CUMULATIVE MATCH DURATION FOR CENTURY (MAY VARY)
ZONE 3	ZONE 5	>2 MINUTES	<10 MINUTES
ZONE 2	ZONE 4	>5 MINUTES	<20 MINUTES
ZONE 1	ZONE 3	>15 MINUTES	<60 MINUTES

can and coasting down the hill. As you begin to slow down at the bottom of the descent to about 40 kph (25 mph), you can begin to pedal again, but not hard. Keep the effort low. You'll be in zone 1. As the speed decreases to 30 kph (19 mph), pedal harder. This should be close to your average speed for the flat sections of the century—within a couple of miles per hour—so your wattage should be what you trained for on flat terrain. That's your base IF.

When speed drops to 20 kph (about 12 mph), you're probably going up a hill. At this point, pedal harder so that your power rises slightly above your normal output on flat terrain. This harder pace is likely one zone above your base IF. On really steep uphills, you'll slow down to around 10 kph (about 6 mph), so here you should pedal quite hard. This is when the match burning kicks in and you're two zones above base IF.

If the speeds I've suggested don't match up with what you expect to do on century day, change them. Instead of 50-40-30-20-10, you may decide to go with 45-35-25-15-5. That would mean 25 kph (15 mph), not 30 kph, is your intended average speed for the century. So you can make slight adjustments to the rule, but the concept remains the same.

Without a doubt, Intensity Factor and Variability Index are the most important predictors of a successful century ride. And, of course, you must take in adequate carbohydrate just as Goldilocks would do—not too much and not too little.

Key and Secondary Workouts

Preparing for a good century takes a lot more than occasionally "going for a ride." Rides must have a purpose, an anticipated benefit; if done frequently enough, they eventually produce a high level of fitness. That is "training."

Some of your workouts when training for a century are more important than others; these are your key workouts. There are also secondary workouts in each period that have slightly less importance. If you divide the last 24 weeks or so of your preparation for the century into two general periods— base and build (as discussed in Chapter 6)—each period has unique key and secondary workouts.

During your key workouts, you must always keep Intensity Factor and Variability Index uppermost in your mind. The single most important workout is the century simulation done in the build period. Your success in the century will come from having rehearsed these two concepts repeatedly on training rides, especially in your training simulations. Riding with an eye on IF and VI must become habitual so that on the Big Day, you do it without even thinking.

Century Simulation and Training Stress

One of the more confounding issues in preparing for a century ride is determining the duration of your long rides. It's not necessary to ride 100 miles in training to prepare for a century. If you do, you will ride at an Intensity Factor well below what you've set for a goal and you'll be on the road for a very long time. As mentioned previously, the key to success for advanced athletes is not duration but intensity. Riding a long time slowly won't get it done.

In the build period, the long rides are your key simulation workouts. You'll probably do 6 to 8 long rides in the final 12 weeks prior to the century, with the last 2 or 3 being the longest. They must all be done at your goal IF, which may involve doing intervals for the higher levels (more on that in a bit). So how long should you make the simulation rides? Table 10.2 will help you to determine the duration of those 2 or 3 longest build-period rides.

Here's how to use Table 10.2 to determine the duration of your 2 or 3 longest key century-simulation rides:

1. Determine your goal century time, taking into account the terrain and any other outside factors (heat, humidity, wind) that may affect your ride.
2. Decide what your goal IF will be for the century. This must be realistic and based on previous performance, in either centuries or long training rides, and the training you have planned.
3. You'll find your projected TSS for the century where the goal time row and IF column intersect (this must be a plain black number—not a number in a gray box or a blank space—to be realistic). More than likely, your TSS should be in the range of 220 to 350.
4. Multiply your projected TSS by 0.75 to determine your longest ride's TSS.
5. Find that longest ride's TSS in your goal IF column; by looking to the time column on the left, you will find your longest ride's duration in preparation for the century.

As mentioned, the duration found using Table 10.2 is what you will do for the last 2 or 3 of your longest rides in the build period. The final one should occur just before you start to taper and peak for the century. (Your taper period begins 2 to 3 weeks prior to the ride; we'll get to it later in this chapter.)

The first of your IF-specific simulation rides in the build period, however, will be much shorter. For most riders, starting out at around 150 TSS is about right. In each week that follows, add 10 percent or so to the previous long ride's TSS. Use TSS to determine how long the ride is—not the other way around. The progression may be something such as 150, 165, 180, 200, and so on until you achieve your goal TSS and long-ride duration as found in Table 10.2. And, of course, all rides must be done at about your goal IF.

TABLE 10.2 ESTIMATED TRAINING STRESS SCORE FOR A CENTURY RIDE BASED ON GOAL INTENSITY FACTOR AND PROJECTED TIME

	0.50 IF	0.55 IF	0.60 IF	0.65 IF	0.70 IF	0.75 IF	0.80 IF
2.75 hours							176
3 hours						169	192
3.25 hours						183	208
3.5 hours					172	197	224
3.75 hours					184	211	240
4 hours				169	196	225	256
4.25 hours				180	208	239	272
4.5 hours				190	221	253	288
4.75 hours			171	201	233	267	304
5 hours			180	211	245	281	320
5.25 hours			189	222	257	295	336
5.5 hours		166	198	232	270	309	352
5.75 hours		174	207	243	282	323	
6 hours	150	182	216	254	294	338	
6.25 hours	156	189	225	264	306	352	
6.5 hours	163	197	234	275	319		
6.75 hours	169	204	243	285	331		
7 hours	175	212	252	296	343		
7.25 hours	181	219	261	306	355		
7.5 hours	188	227	270	317			
7.75 hours	194	234	279	327			
8 hours	200	242	288	338			

NOTE Numbers in gray boxes should not be used.

For some, the goal IF will be too challenging even in a shortened version of what you expect on the day of the century. On that day you'll be well rested, carbohydrate loaded, and eager, and you will have assistance along the way in the form of drafting other riders from time to time and refueling stops. It would be great if all of these were available every time you did a training ride, but that's not going to happen.

Up to an IF of about 0.75, you can expect to ride steadily for several hours on a long training ride. But around and beyond 0.75, it becomes a great challenge to ride for a long time in a workout. That's when you need to include intervals. I recommend zone 3 tempo intervals; you'll find them described in Appendix A. Using intervals, you can simulate the goal IF and get in a long ride. Be sure to pace the intervals by not exceeding the goal IF except on hills. The tendency is to make the first couple of intervals much too hard. Don't do it. Hold back. Pace yourself.

During the long simulation ride, do each thing as closely as you can to the way you expect to do it the day of the event. That includes selecting a similar course, using the same equipment and clothing, and refueling along the way as you will do in the ride itself.

Recovery Workouts

A common way to plan your training week is to alternate hard and easy rides. The hardest rides are the key workouts. The secondary workouts are somewhat easier. Key and secondary workouts can generally be done on back-to-back days by advanced athletes once each week. You will also need days that are intended strictly for recovery. These can be days off the bike with no workout, or they can consist of a short zone 1 ride. A day off once a week is generally a good idea for all riders regardless of ability. Those who are in their first year of serious bike training are best advised to stay off the bike on all recovery days. Research has shown that, whereas advanced athletes recover better with light exercise, novices benefit much more by completely resting.

PREPARING FOR YOUR CENTURY RIDE

Training for a century can't be rushed; you have to plan ahead. In order to develop the appropriate physiological readiness, many changes must take place at the cellular level that simply can't happen quickly, no matter how much you may want them *now*. Trying to force your body to rapidly adapt to hard workouts, such as very high IF combined with very-long-duration rides, almost never works and puts you at great risk. Your body will likely break down in some way with an injury, an illness, burnout, or overtraining. That's its way of saying, "Stop."

The best way to attain readiness for the Big Day is to *gradually* increase the stress over many weeks. Your body will respond positively, and your depth of fitness will be excellent.

In this section we will look at a training progression that works. Training will gradually become more challenging as you progress from the base to the build period and then cap it off with a brief peak period right before your century. I've used this method successfully with many athletes during more than three decades of coaching. I'm sure it will work for you, too.

Base Period

The base period starts some 24 weeks before your century and continues until 12 weeks prior. As described in greater detail in Chapter 6, the purpose of this period is to improve general fitness. For the century rider, that means boosting basic abilities: aerobic endurance, muscular force, speed skills, and muscular endurance.

TABLE 10.3 BASE PERIOD TRAINING ABILITIES WITH ASSOCIATED WORKOUTS IN PARENTHESES FOR THE CENTURY RIDER

PERIOD	KEY WORKOUTS	SECONDARY WORKOUTS
EARLY BASE PERIOD (6–8 WEEKS)	AEROBIC ENDURANCE (AEROBIC THRESHOLD) MUSCULAR FORCE (FORCE REPS)	SPEED SKILLS (DRILLS)
LATE BASE PERIOD (4–6 WEEKS)	MUSCULAR ENDURANCE (SWEET SPOT)	AEROBIC ENDURANCE (AEROBIC THRESHOLD)

See Appendix A for workout details.

Base is divided into early and late subperiods. Early base focuses on developing the first of the three basic abilities. It lasts 6 to 8 weeks, ending when those three, but especially aerobic endurance, are at optimal levels of fitness. See the section "Are You Fitter and Faster?" (page 105) in Chapter 6 for details on how this is determined. The late base period is when the primary focus shifts to muscular endurance. Your goal in this period is to raise your FTP. With consistent training following the schedule presented here, this should happen within 4 to 6 weeks.

Table 10.3 summarizes base period ability training and provides examples of the types of workouts to do for each. The details of the suggested workouts may be found in Appendix A.

Tables 10.4 (early base) and 10.5 (late base) suggest ways to organize your weekly training in order to focus on the key workouts while also fitting in the secondary sessions. These workout schedules are just suggestions and are certainly not the only ways to plan a week's training. Nor are they necessarily the best way for you to do it. You need to create a weekly plan for each period that works for you most of the time. Then dedicate yourself to following it.

TABLE 10.4 A SUGGESTED WEEKLY TRAINING PLAN IN THE EARLY BASE PERIOD FOR THE CENTURY RIDER

DAY	WORKOUT
MONDAY	(DAY OFF FROM TRAINING)
TUESDAY	AEROBIC ENDURANCE
WEDNESDAY	RECOVERY (ZONE 1)
THURSDAY	MUSCULAR FORCE + SPEED SKILLS
FRIDAY	RECOVERY (ZONE 1)
SATURDAY	AEROBIC ENDURANCE
SUNDAY	MUSCULAR FORCE + SPEED SKILLS

See Appendix A for workout details.

TABLE 10.5 A SUGGESTED WEEKLY TRAINING PLAN IN THE LATE BASE PERIOD FOR THE CENTURY RIDER

DAY	WORKOUT
MONDAY	(DAY OFF FROM TRAINING)
TUESDAY	AEROBIC ENDURANCE
WEDNESDAY	MUSCULAR ENDURANCE
THURSDAY	RECOVERY (ZONE 1)
FRIDAY	AEROBIC ENDURANCE
SATURDAY	RECOVERY (ZONE 1)
SUNDAY	MUSCULAR ENDURANCE + AEROBIC ENDURANCE

See Appendix A for workout details.

Your training focus in each week must be on the key workouts. If you have to miss a session due to lifestyle commitments, try to make that missed workout a secondary one. That may mean rearranging the week to fit in all of your key workouts with adequate recovery between them.

TABLE 10.6 BUILD PERIOD TRAINING ABILITIES WITH ASSOCIATED WORKOUTS IN PARENTHESES FOR THE CENTURY RIDER

PERIOD	KEY WORKOUTS	SECONDARY WORKOUTS
BUILD PERIOD (8–9 WEEKS)	MUSCULAR ENDURANCE (CRUISE INTERVALS, FAST GROUP RIDE) CENTURY SIMULATION	AEROBIC ENDURANCE (AEROBIC PACING)

See Appendix A for workout details.

TABLE 10.7 A SUGGESTED WEEKLY TRAINING PLAN IN THE BUILD PERIOD FOR THE CENTURY RIDER

DAY	WORKOUT
MONDAY	(DAY OFF FROM TRAINING)
TUESDAY	MUSCULAR ENDURANCE
WEDNESDAY	RECOVERY (ZONE 1)
THURSDAY	AEROBIC ENDURANCE
FRIDAY	RECOVERY (ZONE 1)
SATURDAY	CENTURY SIMULATION
SUNDAY	RECOVERY

See Appendix A for workout details.

Build Period

The build period starts 12 weeks before your century and lasts for 9 or 10 weeks. During this time, the focus of training is on becoming faster. That includes terrain familiarization, event nutrition, pacing rehearsal, and equipment selection. It also means maintaining the aerobic endurance gains made in the base period while improving event-specific fitness. The most important weekly workout now is the century-simulation ride described above.

Table 10.6 lays out the key and secondary workouts for the build period. A suggested weekly training plan is provided in Table 10.7. Note here that I've put the long, simulation ride on Saturday. It's there for a reason: Should Saturday turn out to be a foul-weather day, you can still do your long ride on Sunday.

Peaking for a Century

The last 2 to 3 weeks before your century is the time to start your taper in order to peak by coming into form. This is the peak period. Form results from reducing the duration and frequency of the workouts while maintaining intensity. The interplay among Chronic Training Load (CTL), Acute Training Load (ATL), and Training Stress Balance (TSB), explained in Chapter 7, is key to the shift to the peak period. It may be helpful at this point to reread the section "Power and Periodization" (page 125) in that chapter to refresh your memory on the details of coming into form.

A quick summary of peaking is that you are attempting to raise your TSB (form) while at the same time reducing ATL (fatigue). This is accomplished by gradually reducing your daily and weekly TSS throughout the 2- to 3-week peak period. By reducing the duration and frequency of your key workouts, you'll decrease your TSS. You will lose a little bit of fitness, but you will also shed a great deal of fatigue. As a result, you will come into form. You'll be race ready.

Using the calendar function on WKO+ software or online at Training-Peaks.com, you can manage and even predict your TSB on century day by projecting what your daily TSS will be for every day in the peak period. The Performance Management Chart then shows the results. Figure 10.1 is such a chart showing a projected peak period using the training methodology described above. It illustrates how TSB rises as CTL slightly falls throughout a 2-week peak period.

For the day of your century, you want "strong form." That means CTL (fitness) has only decreased about 10 percent or less from the start of the

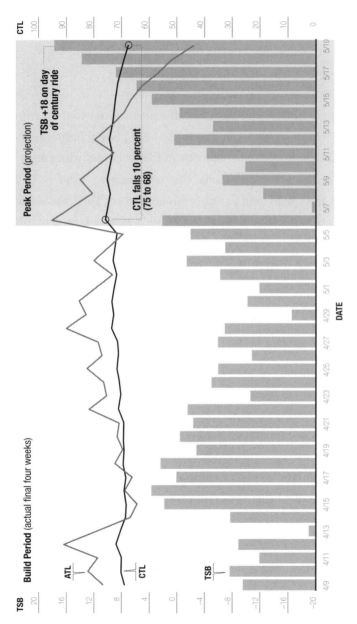

FIGURE 10.1 Performance Management Chart showing a projected peak period ending on the day of a century

peak period 2 to 3 weeks prior to the event and TSB (form) has risen into the range of +15 to +25. "Weak form" may still produce an in-range TSB, although it's usually much too high, but fitness will drop by more than 10 percent. If the prediction on your Performance Management Chart shows that CTL and TSB are not where you want them on the day of your century, you should simply plug in new projections for daily TSS numbers until CTL and TSB are correct. Then do the workouts each day that produce the projected TSS or something quite close.

The key workouts during the peak period are century-simulation rides. But they are much shorter than what you've been doing throughout the build period. TSS, rather than time, is used to determine how long each ride lasts. So pay attention to this field on your head unit while riding. The real key for these workouts is Intensity Factor, not duration. Again, you're reducing only duration and frequency in order to shed fatigue (ATL). If you also reduce the IF of the simulation rides, fatigue will be lost too quickly and you'll wind up with weak form.

Do one of these simulation rides every third day, with recovery workouts between them. Table 10.8 suggests a training plan for the first 2 weeks of a 3-week peak period. Should you decide to taper for only 2 weeks, omit the first week here and start with the second week. Short tapers are used when training has not gone well in the build period and another week of high-TSS training is needed.

Tables 10.9 and 10.10 offer suggested plans for the week that culminates with your century. The workouts and their patterns are significantly different from what you did in the previous weeks of the peak period. Daily TSS is reduced even more as IF stays high by doing intervals or hill repeats at the highest intensity expected for the century. The hills should be quite short, taking only about 90 seconds to climb. This reflects the 50-40-30-20-10 Rule

TABLE 10.8 A SUGGESTED TRAINING PLAN FOR THE FIRST 2 WEEKS OF A 3-WEEK PEAK PERIOD FOR A CENTURY RIDER

WEEK 1	WORKOUT
MONDAY	CENTURY SIMULATION (80–100 TSS) (IF PREVIOUS SUNDAY'S WORKOUT WAS A SIMULATION, TAKE TODAY OFF.)
TUESDAY	RECOVERY (ZONE 1, 30–50 TSS)
WEDNESDAY	RECOVERY (ZONE 1, 30–50 TSS)
THURSDAY	CENTURY SIMULATION (90–120 TSS)
FRIDAY	RECOVERY (ZONE 1, 30–50 TSS)
SATURDAY	RECOVERY (ZONE 1, 30–50 TSS)
SUNDAY	CENTURY SIMULATION (150–250 TSS)
WEEK 2	**WORKOUT**
MONDAY	RECOVERY (ZONE 1, 30–50 TSS)
TUESDAY	RECOVERY (ZONE 1, 30–50 TSS)
WEDNESDAY	CENTURY SIMULATION (80–110 TSS)
THURSDAY	RECOVERY (ZONE 1, 30–50 TSS)
FRIDAY	RECOVERY (ZONE 1, 30–50 TSS)
SATURDAY	CENTURY SIMULATION (100–120 TSS)
SUNDAY	RECOVERY (ZONE 1, 30–50 TSS)

TABLE 10.9 SUGGESTED LAST WEEK OF A 2- OR 3-WEEK PEAK PERIOD FOR A CENTURY RIDE ON A SATURDAY

WEEK 3	WORKOUT
MONDAY	RECOVERY (ZONE 1, 20–30 TSS) OR DAY OFF
TUESDAY	SHORT RIDE WITH 4 × 90-SECOND HILL REPEATS AT CENTURY IF (50–60 TSS)
WEDNESDAY	SHORT RIDE WITH 3 × 90-SECOND HILL REPEATS AT CENTURY IF (40–50 TSS)
THURSDAY	RECOVERY (ZONE 1, 20–30 TSS) OR DAY OFF
FRIDAY	SHORT RIDE WITH 1 × 90-SECOND HILL CLIMB AT CENTURY IF (20–30 TSS)
SATURDAY	CENTURY RIDE
SUNDAY	DAY OFF

TABLE 10.10 SUGGESTED LAST WEEK OF A 2- OR 3-WEEK PEAK PERIOD FOR A CENTURY RIDE ON A SUNDAY	
WEEK 3	**WORKOUT**
MONDAY	RECOVERY (ZONE 1, 20–30 TSS) OR DAY OFF
TUESDAY	SHORT RIDE WITH 5 × 90-SECOND HILL REPEATS AT CENTURY IF (50–60 TSS)
WEDNESDAY	RECOVERY (ZONE 1, 20–30 TSS)
THURSDAY	SHORT RIDE WITH 3 × 90-SECOND HILL REPEATS AT CENTURY IF (40–50 TSS)
FRIDAY	RECOVERY (ZONE 1, 20–30 TSS) OR DAY OFF
SATURDAY	SHORT RIDE WITH 1 × 90-SECOND HILL CLIMB AT CENTURY IF (20–30 TSS)
SUNDAY	CENTURY RIDE

and steady-state match burning discussed earlier in this chapter. Note that Table 10.9 is for a Saturday event; 10.10 is for a Sunday century.

PREPARING FOR A CENTURY is a challenging task even for advanced and experienced riders. Once you've developed general fitness in the base period, the keys to century success are getting the Variability Index and Intensity Factor right for the long simulation rides in the build period. Determining the duration of those longest weekly rides is another challenge made much easier by your power meter and analysis software. By customizing the power-based weekly training plans suggested in this chapter to fit your unique needs, you will come into strong form at the right time and have an excellent century ride.

APPENDIX A

POWER-BASED WORKOUTS

The following workouts are categorized by training ability, as described in Chapter 4. These represent only a few of many possibilities. For more examples, see *The Cyclist's Training Bible*, *The Triathlete's Training Bible*, or *The Mountain Biker's Training Bible*. The web site TrainingPeaks.com also provides hundreds of my workouts in a menu format.

For the advanced rider, workouts may be combined to form longer sessions. Combinations are most commonly done in the build period. For example, after warming up, a road cyclist may start with anaerobic endurance intervals followed by muscular endurance intervals and then finish with power sprint training. A triathlete may start with aerobic threshold and then do cruise intervals followed by aerobic pacing. The purpose of combining workouts is to make the session more racelike.

A proper warm-up before starting the workout is assumed and so is not included in the descriptions that follow.

Aerobic Endurance Workouts

Aerobic threshold. Ride steadily in the lower half of heart rate zone 2 (using the Friel heart rate zone system; see Appendix B). See your sport-specific chapter (8, 9, or 10) for the duration of this ride. Power may vary during the ride. That's acceptable so long as heart rate stays in the proper range.

In the post-ride analysis, check your Variability Index, Efficiency Factor, and decoupling. The purpose of this workout is to improve aerobic endurance.

Aerobic pacing. Ride steadily in power zone 2 for a race-appropriate duration. This is typically 2 or more hours. Rehearse the use of the 50-40-30-20-10 Rule and proper use of your steady-state matches on hills.

In the post-ride analysis, check your Variability Index, Efficiency Factor, and decoupling. The purpose of this workout is to maintain aerobic endurance.

Muscular Force Workouts

Force reps. These may be done on a hill or on flat terrain. Select a high gear (such as 53×14), and then coast to a near stop at the base of the hill or the start point for the repetition. While seated, drive the pedals down with great force. Do only 6 to 12 pedal revolutions (count 1 leg only) for each repetition. Your cadence will be very slow at first, well under 50 rpm, and will increase as you progress through the 6 to 12 revolutions.

Power should peak at a high level. Strive for a Peak Power on each of at least double your FTP. Do 1 to 3 sets of 3 repetitions in a workout.

Recover in zone 1 for 3 minutes after each repetition and for 6 minutes between sets.

The risk of injury, especially to the knees, is high for this workout. Stop the workout at the first sign of unusual joint discomfort. The purpose of this workout is to increase muscular force production.

Speed Skills Workouts

High-cadence drill. There are many drills to improve pedaling skills; this is the most common and basic.

In the course of a given workout of your choice, insert several high-cadence intervals of a few minutes each. During each of these intervals, increase your cadence to a level that is just slightly uncomfortable and then maintain it for the length of the interval. Use a low (easy) gear.

Recover between intervals for several minutes while pedaling at your normal cadence.

Over the course of several weeks, extend the duration of each interval and the combined interval time for the workout. The purpose of this workout is to improve pedaling efficiency.

Muscular Endurance Workouts

Sweet-spot intervals. These intervals are best done on a flat course or one that has a slight uphill grade. Complete 2 intervals of 20 minutes each at an Intensity Factor of 0.88 to 0.93. Recover in zone 1 for 5 minutes between intervals.

The first few times you do this workout within a block of training, you may find it helpful to start with shorter intervals by doing something such as 4 × 10 minutes with 2.5-minute recoveries in zone 1 or 3 × 15 minutes with 4-minute recoveries. The purpose of this workout is to increase your Functional Threshold Power.

Cruise intervals. These may be done on flat terrain or up a hill similar to what is expected in your race. Do 3 to 5 intervals of 5 to 12 minutes each at an intensity equal to power zone 4. The recoveries between the intervals are in power zone 1 and are about a fourth as long as the preceding interval. For example, if an interval is 6 minutes long, the recovery following it is 90 seconds. A 12-minute interval would be followed by a 3-minute recovery.

Cruise intervals performed on a hill may make it impossible to keep the recoveries to a fourth of the interval duration due to the time required to descend. In this case, return to the bottom of the hill and start the next interval as soon as possible. The purpose of this workout is to improve muscular endurance.

Tempo intervals. This workout is best done on a course that simulates your racecourse. Complete several intervals of 20 minutes each at power zone 3. The number of intervals you should do depends on the event for which you are training. A criterium racer may do 3, whereas an Ironman triathlete or century rider may do 6 to 8.

Recover by pedaling easily in power zone 1 for 5 minutes after each interval.

Use a small number of intervals the first few times you do this workout in a block of training. Increase the number of intervals with each subsequent session or two. Be sure to practice your pacing strategy (50-40-30-20-10 Rule and match-burning control). The purpose of this workout is to improve muscular endurance.

Anaerobic Endurance Workouts

Fast group ride. For the road cyclist, this is the ultimate race-simulation workout in the build period. In order to simulate the anticipated Training Stress Score of a road race, however, it's possible that that the entire ride may need to be longer than the group-ride portion. It's common, therefore, to precede or follow the group ride with race-appropriate intervals. The purpose of this workout is to prepare for a road race or criterium.

VO_2max intervals. These intervals may be done on flat terrain or on a hill. Do 3 to 8 intervals of 2 to 4 minutes each in power zone 5. It's common to do 8 to 20 minutes of total interval time within such a workout.

Recover in zone 1 for the same amount of time as the previous interval.

This is a high-risk workout. Be aware of joint discomfort, especially the knees. Safety must also be a concern when doing this workout on the open road. Find a stretch of road where there are no intersections and the traffic is light. The purpose of this workout is to boost aerobic capacity or prepare for the stresses of a road race or criterium.

Match-burning intervals. Complete several sets of short intervals with brief and incomplete recoveries (in zone 1) between them. Group the intervals by sets with longer recoveries (on the order of 2 to 5 minutes) between sets. How long each interval lasts, how great the power is, and how many such intervals you do in a session depend on your definition of a "match" (see Chapter 5 for details) and what you anticipate the demands of your race will be.

A typical road race workout is 3 sets of 5 intervals with each interval in zone 6 and lasting 20 to 30 seconds. The recoveries may be 40 to 50 seconds between intervals and 3 minutes between sets. Your purpose in doing this workout is to prepare for the high-intensity matches that determine the outcomes of criteriums and road races.

Sprint Power Workouts

Jumps. During an otherwise moderate- to low-intensity ride, include several very brief all-out sprints lasting perhaps 6 to 8 pedal strokes each.

Do these on varied terrain: flat, uphill, and downhill. Also do them both in and out of the saddle. Include some sprints holding on to the brake hoods and others while in the drops. Cadence should be high.

Between sprints, return to the workout's general intensity (such as zone 2), taking a long time to recover between sprints.

This workout is often best done with a training partner for head-to-head competition. The purpose is to achieve as high a wattage as possible in the shortest amount of time.

Hill sprints. On to a hill with a 4 to 6 percent grade, do 6 to 9 sprints. Use a flying start for each sprint, taking several seconds to build speed on the approach to the hill. Sprint up the hill for 10 to 15 pedal strokes at maximal effort with a high cadence.

Recover for 3 to 6 minutes after each sprint. The purpose of this workout is to increase sprint power.

APPENDIX B

SETTING HEART RATE ZONES FOR CYCLING

This quick guide will help you get the intensity of your workouts dialed in for your heart rate monitor. Note that the lactate threshold heart rate test is best done early in the base and build periods.

Step 1. Determine your lactate threshold heart rate (LTHR) with the following short test. (Do not use 220 minus your age to find max heart rate, as this is as likely to be wrong as right. For a deeper explanation, see my book *Total Heart Rate Training.*)

To find your LTHR, do a 30-minute time trial all by yourself (no training partners and not in a race). This time trial should be ridden as if it were a race for the entire 30 minutes. At 10 minutes into the test, click the lap button on your heart rate monitor. When done, check the monitor display for your average heart rate for the last 20 minutes. That number is an approximation of your LTHR.

Note: I am frequently asked if you should go hard for the first 10 minutes. The answer is yes. Go hard for the entire 30 minutes. But be aware that most people doing this test go too hard the first few minutes and then gradually slow down for the remainder. Doing so will give you inaccurate results. The more times you do this test, the more accurate your LTHR is likely to become, as you will learn to pace yourself better at the start.

Step 2. Establish your training zones using the following guide:

ZONE 1	Less than 81% of LTHR
ZONE 2	81% to 89% of LTHR
ZONE 3	90% to 93% of LTHR
ZONE 4	94% to 99% of LTHR
ZONE 5A	100% to 102% of LTHR
ZONE 5B	103% to 106% of LTHR
ZONE 5C	More than 106% of LTHR

APPENDIX C

ANALYSIS SOFTWARE

At the time of publication, eight software products were available for use with power meter head units. The prices listed here were correct at the time but may have since changed. For the most current information, check the product's web site and read all details before purchasing. Be sure to check whether the software is compatible with your head unit and desktop computer (as applicable).

GoldenCheetah (goldencheetah.org). This is a free, open-source software product that continues to be refined by dedicated programmers who donate their time. It's compatible with Mac, Windows, and Linux computer operating systems. You can download an SRM or PowerTap directly to it.

Polar Precision Performance (polar.fi/en/support/downloads?product). If you use a Polar power device, use this software for setup and analysis. Polar Precision Performance is available as a free download.

PowerAgent (cycleops.com/products/software.html). If you have a Power-Tap power meter, you will need to use this free software, which comes with it, to configure the head unit. You can use it as well as other software for analysis.

PowerCoach (powercoach.ch). This software has a broad range of usage. It is compatible with Windows and Mac computers and comes in English,

French, and German versions. PowerCoach can be used in conjunction with iBike, Garmin, Polar, PowerTap, and SRM head units. It costs $750 online.

RaceDay Apollo (physfarm.com/inside/raceday.html). Apollo can be used with iBike, Garmin, Polar, PowerTap, and SRM devices, and it operates on Mac and Windows computer systems. It sells for a onetime fee of $125.

SRM Win (srm.de/us/software). This software comes in the box with an SRM power meter but may also be downloaded for free. It provides many analysis functions. If you have an SRM, you will need to use this to program your device, but other software may be used for SRM analysis.

TrainingPeaks (trainingpeaks.com). This is the only online software currently available for power meter users. It may also be used with a wide range of other products, such as heart rate monitors, GPS watches, accelerometers, basic handlebar computers, and mapping devices. The features and displays are quite robust and similar to WKO+. Data stored here from any power meter may be easily accessed by your coach, who can then analyze it for you. As a user you pay a subscription fee of about $20 per month.

WKO+ (trainingpeaks.com/wko). WKO+ ("workout plus") is compatible with all available power meters as well as a wide range of device types, such as heart rate monitors, GPS watches, and accelerometers. All downloaded data can be uploaded to the user's TrainingPeaks account for backup. WKO+ is not compatible with Mac computers, but third-party software that converts Windows to Mac enables use on the Mac platform. It costs $129. There is a free 14-day trial period so that you can see if you like the software before purchase.

GLOSSARY

5 Percent Rule. A rule according to which, when the duration of the session or a segment thereof doubles, the power to ride at a maximal effort for the longer duration decreases by 5 percent.

50-40-30-20-10 Rule. A rule that assists with pacing based on a combination of speed and effort.

Acute Training Load (ATL). The recent workload of training (such as past 7 days) as defined by frequency, intensity, and duration. Expressed as Training Stress Score per day.

Aerobic threshold. A zone 2 workout aimed at boosting aerobic endurance.

Average power. The total amount of power data collected during a ride divided by the number of time units (minutes, for example) during which it was collected.

Bottom bracket. A housing or support for the ball bearing races for the cranks through which the cranks are connected, found at the intersection of the seat tube, down tube, and chainstays on a bicycle.

Cadence. The rate at which pedals are turned on a bicycle. See "Revolutions per minute."

Chronic Training Load (CTL). The workload of a relatively long period of training (such as 6 weeks) as defined by frequency, intensity, and duration. Expressed as Training Stress Score per day.

Crank arms. The extensions from the bottom bracket of the bike to which the pedals are attached.

Cruise intervals. An interval workout done in zone 4.

Fast Find. A function in WKO+ software and on TrainingPeaks.com that allows the user to find specific intensities often referred to as "matches."

Force. To overcome resistance, as in pushing down on the pedal. See "Torque."

Force reps. A workout done with very brief repetitions at maximal power in a high gear with a low cadence with the intent of improving muscular force.

Functional Threshold Power (FTP). The highest mean maximal power a rider can sustain for 60 minutes.

Intensity Factor (IF). The ratio of a rider's Normalized Power to Functional Threshold Power. An indicator of how challenging the workout or segment thereof was in terms of intensity only.

Jumps. A workout with several short, maximal-effort sprints intended to improve sprint power.

Key workout. A workout designed to prepare a rider for the specific demands of the event for which she or he is training.

KiloCalorie. Usually referred to as "calories," the unit of measurement for biological energy expended while riding a bike. See "kiloJoule."

KiloJoule (kJ). The unit of measurement for mechanical energy (1 kiloCalorie = 4.184 kiloJoules).

Lactate threshold. The intensity at which the blood lactate level first begins to exceed lactate removal.

Match. A relatively brief effort during a race performed at an intensity that cannot be maintained for very long given the nature of the race but that may be necessary for competitive purposes.

Normalized Power (NP). An expression of average power adjusted for the range of variability of power during a ride. A better reflection of the metabolic cost ("kiloCalories") and effort of a ride than "average power."

Peak Power. The highest average power a rider can achieve for a given unit of time, such as 1 minute, 5 minutes, or 60 minutes.

Performance Management Chart. An analysis tool available in WKO+ software and at TrainingPeaks.com that allows the user to monitor and manage Chronic Training Load, Acute Training Load, and Training Stress Balance.

Power. In physics, the result of force and velocity. In cycling, the result of rotational force (torque) and pedal cadence.

Power meter. In cycling, a device that measures torque and pedal cadence in order to measure and display power.

Power Profile. A chart that graphically shows the best Peak Power levels across a wide spectrum of durations.

Rating of perceived exertion (RPE). A subjective scoring of the effort a rider is experiencing at a given moment in time. Usually expressed on a 0–10 or 6–20 scale.

Revolutions per minute (RPM). The number of pedal strokes completed in 1 minute. See "Cadence."

Strain gauge. A device built into a power meter that measures electrical resistance as the result of shape change due to the application of force.

Sweet spot. A segment of a workout done at 88 to 93 percent of Functional Threshold Power.

Tapering. A training model in which the training workload is decreased over a period of several days in order to peak for an event.

Tempo. A workout done in zone 3.

Torque. In cycling, a rotational force applied to crank arms.

Training Stress Score (TSS). The workload of a training session based on intensity and duration.

Variability Index (VI). The ratio of Normalized Power to average power for a ride. Closely associated with pacing.

Velocity. Distance divided by time. Speed.

VO$_2$max intervals. An interval workout done in power zone 5.

Watt. The unit of measure for power.

Work. The moving of an object through a distance.

ACKNOWLEDGMENTS

First I want to thank the many athletes I have coached who have allowed me to try out new ideas with their training while my knowledge of power-based cycling developed over the past 15 years. Without their trust in my way of doing things, this book never would have happened. Thank you!

I especially want to thank Dr. Andrew Coggan for his groundbreaking work, which has largely defined what training and racing with power are all about. He quickly brought a relatively new technology into the computer age with his insightful analysis. Much of this book is based on his model. I continue to be in awe of all he has done for power-based training in such a short time.

There are many others who have contributed to this book's development from an outline to what you now hold in your hands. A heartfelt "thank you" goes out to all of the following.

Hunter Allen for his and Dr. Coggan's book, *Training and Racing with a Power Meter*, which initially guided me through most of the details of power-based training and which I highly recommend to all cyclists. Theirs is by far the most comprehensive description of the topic.

Bill Cofer, my friend of 41 years and occasional training partner, for offering enthusiastic and detailed help with an explanation of the physics of power in Chapter 2 and his suggestions for Chapter 10.

Ted Costantino, publisher of VeloPress, for providing guidance on the many issues I faced in writing this, for keeping me on track throughout the writing process, and for solving my many challenges in explaining complex concepts.

Exercise physiologist Alan Couzens for his input on speed relative to power in pacing with his 50-40-30-20-10 Rule.

Gear Fisher, the CEO of Peaksware, LLC, for assisting with power analysis software terminology.

Dirk Friel, my son, for reviewing software graphics and for helping on the sections dealing with handlebar computers.

Justin Henkel, the director of education for Saris, for suggesting this book and helping to define its purpose.

Renee Jardine of VeloPress for giving the book its initial form, voice, and focus and for continuing to support my ideas for book projects.

Uli Schoberer, the inventor of the first mobile power meter and the owner of SRM, for lending me a power meter to try in 1995 and thus initiating my interest in power-based training.

Finally, I want to thank Joyce, my supportive and loving wife of 46 years, for encouraging and assisting with my sometimes quirky ideas. She continues to be there for me despite my 4:00 a.m. wake-ups as I study and write about things that interest me.

INDEX

watts per kilogram of body weight display (W/KG), 39
Heart rate, 9, 10
    disconnection from performance (output), 11, 16–17
    display (HR), 36
    effect of hill climb on, 14–16, 15f.
    as measure of input, 16–17
    "outside" forces affecting, 11
    and power, 46–47

Input, 93
    heart rate and RPE as measures of, 16–17
Intensity, 72, 120, 155
    and warm-up, 155
Intensity Factor (IF), 71, 72, 73–74
    and build period, 101
    and century rides, 192–193
    common ones, 73t.
    display, 39
    and FTP, 72–73
    and recovery workouts, 153–154
    and triathlons, 167–169
    and triathlon-specific workout, 103–105
Ironman, and economy, 31

KiloJoules, 40–41
    per hour, display (KJ/HR), 39

Lactate Threshold (zone 4), 52, 63t. *See also* Anaerobic threshold
Lactate threshold heart rate (LTHR), 52–53
Left-right pedal balance display (L-R), 39

Mashers, 32
Matches, 71
    defined, 85–86, 88
    and steady-state races, 88–89, 88t., 146
    and training for road racing, 160
    using Fast Find in WKO+, 86, 87f.
    and variably paced races, 84–86
Multisystem training, 14–16
Muscles
    as focus of training, 10
    type 1 (slow-twitch), 27

type 2 (fast-twitch), 27
type 2a, 27–28
type 2x, 28
Muscular endurance workouts, 66–67, 150–151, 179
Muscular force workouts, 65–66, 158, 179

Normalized power, 42–44, 94, 96
    display (NORM PWR), 39

Output, 93
    power as measure of, 16–17
    speed as measure of, 16–17

Pacing, 71
Pacing
    and acidosis, 78–79
    and 50-40-30-20-10 Rule, 83–84, 83t., 145–146, 168, 195–196
    and glycogen, 77–79
    in road races, 142–144, 144f., 145f.
    steadily paced races, 81–84
    in time trials, 145–146
    and triathlons, 167–169
    and Variability Index (VI), 79–81, 80f., 81f.
Peak power, 74
    monitoring changes in, 110–112, 111f., 112f.
    profiling, 71, 74, 75–77, 75f., 76f.
    and road races, 141–142
Peaking, 131
Performance
    defined, 3
    increasing, 4
Performance Management Chart, 126, 127f.
    and form, 131–135, 134f.
    in managing fitness and fatigue, 128–130, 130f., 131f.
Power
    average, 41
    in cycling, 24–25
    display (WATTS or PWR), 36
    and duration, 74
    effect of hill climb on, 14–16, 15f.

ABOUT THE AUTHOR

JOE FRIEL is the cofounder of TrainingPeaks.com and TrainingBible Coaching. With a master of science degree in exercise science, he has an extensive background in coaching, having trained endurance athletes since 1980. His clients have included novices, elite amateurs, and professionals. The list includes an Ironman Triathlon winner, USA and foreign national champions, world championship competitors, and an Olympian.

Joe is the author of several books, including *The Cyclist's Training Bible, The Triathlete's Training Bible, The Mountain Biker's Training Bible, Cycling Past 50, Your First Triathlon, Your Best Triathlon,* and *Total Heart Rate Training,* and coauthor of *Going Long, The Paleo Diet for Athletes, Precision Heart Rate Training,* and *Triathlon Science.*

He has been a columnist for *Inside Triathlon, VeloNews,* and *220* magazines, and he frequently writes articles for other international magazines and web sites. He conducts seminars and camps for endurance athletes and provides consulting services to corporations and to national governing bodies.

As an age-group competitor, he is a former Colorado State Masters Triathlon Champion and a Rocky Mountain region and Southwest region duathlon age-group champion. He has been named to several All-American teams and has represented the United States at world championships. He also competes in USA Cycling bike races and time trials.

Joe Friel may be contacted through his blog at joefrielsblog.com.

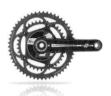
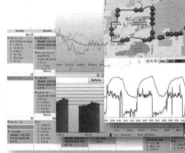
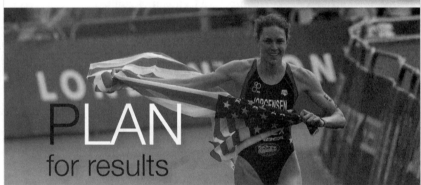